HEALTHY *for* LIFE

FOUNDATIONAL SKILLS FOR PARENTS, TEACHERS, MENTORS, AND THE KIDS THEY LOVE

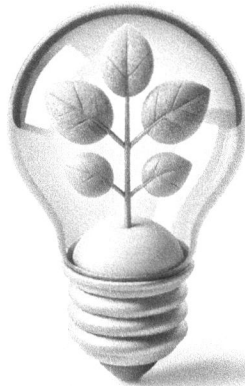

ILANA ZABLOZKI-AMIR, MD

Featuring: Dr. Bo Babenko • Monique Bogni • Gina Bria • Philippe Brouillard
Sandra Cammarata, MD • Giovanni Campanile, MD • Dr. Amanda A. Carpenter
Amy Levine Cohen • Dr. Stephen Cohen • Stephen Dahmer, MD • Emily Givler
Maryann Herklotz • Dr. Najwa Bahsoun Jaber • Eyal Levit, MD
Francesca MacDonald • Michael MacDonald • Patrick J. Nardulli
Laurel Parker-Chan • Mariah Ramundo • Dr. Elina K. Restrepo
Dr. Adria Rothfeld • Dr. Heather Schuerlein • Caitilin Twain • Marina Vaysbaum

HEALTHY *for* LIFE

FOUNDATIONAL SKILLS FOR PARENTS, TEACHERS, MENTORS, AND THE KIDS THEY LOVE

ILANA ZABLOZKI-AMIR, MD

Featuring: Dr. Bo Babenko • Monique Bogni • Gina Bria • Philippe Brouillard
Sandra Cammarata, MD • Giovanni Campanile, MD • Dr. Amanda A. Carpenter
Amy Levine Cohen • Dr. Stephen Cohen • Stephen Dahmer, MD • Emily Givler
Maryann Herklotz • Dr. Najwa Bahsoun Jaber • Eyal Levit, MD
Francesca MacDonald • Michael MacDonald • Patrick J. Nardulli
Laurel Parker-Chan • Mariah Ramundo • Dr. Elina K. Restrepo
Dr. Adria Rothfeld • Dr. Heather Schuerlein • Caitilin Twain • Marina Vaysbaum

DEDICATION

I dedicate this book to:

My three sons, Alexander, Jonathan, and Jorden. You are my inspirations for this book! When you were little and always at home, I tried to guide you as best I could to make the healthiest and safest choices. And our environment was set up to support that. But now you're adults living in a world that's not always looking out for your best interests, even though it pretends to. I hope everything I taught you and the habits you've grown with continue to guide you through. But there's way more to know and encounter!

I hope with all my heart that you'll consistently prioritize the foundations of health—the pillars in this book. There is amazing wisdom here, with skills to keep building on. You know some of the authors in this book well, and you know they are my go-to's for anything health-related. Now we have even more. Thank you for your trust in me. I love you!

The memory of my father, Alexander "Sasha" Zablozki. His story was the catalyst for my story. And every single day, what I do is in his honor.

My mom Dr. Vera Zablozki. Mommy, you are the greatest person I know. I could never have accomplished what I have—personally and professionally—without your unconditional love, support, wisdom, intelligence, energy, proactivity, encouragement, and so much more. xoxo

My husband Mark. There is no one in this world who could be a more perfect person to navigate life with. How lucky I am to have someone who always lovingly encourages me to do my thing. And everything I do is better when you're by my side. xoxo

DISCLAIMER

This book is designed to provide competent, reliable, and educational information regarding health and wellness and other subject matter covered. However, it is sold with the understanding the authors and publisher specifically disclaim all responsibility for any liability, loss, or risk, personal or otherwise, incurred as a consequence, directly or indirectly, of the use and application of any of the contents of this publication.

In order to maintain the anonymity of others, the names and identifying characteristics of some people, places, and organizations described in this book may have been changed.

This publication contains content that may be potentially triggering or disturbing. Individuals who are sensitive to certain themes are advised to exercise caution while reading.

The opinions, ideas, and recommendations contained in this publication do not necessarily represent those of the publisher or the individual authors. The use of any information provided in this book is solely at your own risk.

Our authors represent cultures worldwide and as such, there may be differences in language and expressions. As a global publisher, we have made the conscious choice to not edit these nuances so each chapter is authentic and in its author's words.

Know that the experts here have shared their tools, practices, and knowledge with you with a sincere and generous intent to assist you on your health and wellness journey. Please contact them with any questions you may have about the techniques or information they provided. They will be happy to assist you further and be an ongoing resource for your success!

TABLE OF CONTENTS

PILLAR 3
REGULATION OF
THE NERVOUS SYSTEM | 159

INTRODUCTION

As I sat in the dental chair, fresh from a teeth cleaning, the faint sound of papers rustling caught my attention. Through the open door, I could hear the dentist flipping through my chart, likely reviewing my records before stepping in. Moments later, she entered with a warm smile and the standard pleasantries, asking how I was doing.

It had been years since my last visit with her, yet she remembered—"Oh yes, you're a physician," she said, her eyes lighting up, "a holistic one." I could almost see the gears turning in her head as she reached for her tools. Then, she paused.

"Can I ask you something?" She hesitated for a second. "My husband's cholesterol is high. What supplements should he take?"

Now, your first thought may be: *Good question—I want to know, too!* Or *Seriously? This isn't really the time and place for that kind of question.*

My first thought came with an emphatic chuckle—the dentist's question was one I hear often, from friends, family, even strangers who discover my line of work. My next thought was: *Oh boy, her mind is on something else as she is about to put these metal tools in my mouth.*

Respectfully, I replied, "It depends." I didn't have a one-size-fits-all answer. How could I, without knowing his full health history, lifestyle, and the root causes of his high cholesterol? As I watched her thoughtful nod, I felt a pang of sadness. Here she was, a highly trained professional, yet so unsure and searching for answers that should already be embedded in our healthcare system.

Why is it that, despite all the technological advancements, we still don't know how to prevent or effectively address chronic conditions and spiraling health trajectories?

We didn't talk much more about it, and I got a clean bill of health, at least for my mouth. But I left with a nagging feeling.

It's no secret that our healthcare system, while brilliant at managing acute crises, is reactive at best when it comes to long-term wellness. We excel at life-saving surgeries, groundbreaking medications, and cutting-edge technologies, but when it comes to preventing chronic conditions and teaching people how to live truly healthy lives, we fall short.

Doctors, in general, aren't trained to prioritize the core foundations of health—*nutrition, environmental exposures, stress management, fitness, and sleep.* These pillars, which I call the *"forgotten foundations,"* are the bedrock of sustainable well-being, yet they're largely absent from medical school curricula.

This educational gap continues through residency, medical conferences, and mentorships, where, commonly, the focus remains on diagnosing and treating symptoms, rather than addressing root causes. As a result, these essential aspects of health are often glossed over or outright ignored. Even more concerning, alternative therapies that could offer meaningful benefits are often dismissed without being given proper consideration.

This reactive approach to health becomes a self-perpetuating cycle, with few professionals questioning it. Meanwhile, insurance companies often control which diagnostic evaluations and treatments are approved and even how much time doctors can spend with each patient. When the system prioritizes cost control over patient-centered care, the outcome is what we see today: a reactive healthcare model that fails millions.

This is why I felt compelled to spearhead this book. People are taking health into their own hands —which is a great thing. The problem is that we're frequently bombarded with conflicting or misleading information. For example, one source might claim that a certain food is the key to longevity, while another warns it could be dangerous to one's health. And it wouldn't be unusual to find these dueling claims side by side on a web search. It's hard to know whom or what to trust.

Even when people do find accurate information, there's often a disconnect between knowledge and action. Having the right information is one thing, but understanding how to implement it in a sustainable, meaningful way is another. This is where so many people get stuck—feeling overwhelmed by the sheer volume of advice and unsure of how to make it work in their own lives, let alone for their children or the people they care for. This is why it makes good sense and can be so impactful to begin with one small, manageable change, model it, teach it, and then gradually build on it. And when you teach your kids from a young age, the easier it is for habits and skills to become more deeply ingrained.

So welcome to *Healthy for Life*! Consider it your framework for Proactive Health.

Proactive health is about being intentional and strategic with your health choices in order to build resilience, strengthen the body's systems, and maintain optimal functioning. It's about doing what you can, starting as early as you can, to keep healthy and vibrant for as long as possible.

I often say to people: "There are lots of simple things you can do for your health! But keeping healthy isn't always so simple." **The key is to understand the foundations of what the body needs, no matter the health circumstance or goal, and to develop a diverse go-to skill set that lets you readily implement them in your life.**

When it comes to health, our society's current priorities are far from user-friendly, and they create significant obstacles to self-care. With rampant advertising of highly processed foods that are way too high in sugar and low in nutritional value while being disguised as "fun food," it's all too easy to choose convenience over health. And we're a culture that glorifies constant productivity, often leaving little room for rest and recovery, leading to chronic fatigue and burnout. The presence of harmful chemicals in our food, water, and environment poses further risks, making it even more challenging to keep our "threat buckets" from overflowing.

The term *threat bucket* refers to the cumulative impact of various risks on our health. Each harmful exposure adds to this bucket, and when it overflows, it can lead to serious health issues. I firmly believe that by making self-care simpler and resources more accessible, we can create a lasting shift in the healthcare system—one that will have ripple effects for generations to come.

THE FIVE PILLARS: THE CORE FOUNDATIONS OF HEALTH

1. **Nutrition**
2. **Environment**
3. **Regulation of the Nervous System**
4. **Fitness and Movement**
5. **Sleep, Repair, and Recharge**

You can remember the pillars with the acronym N.E.R.F.S. You'll learn more about each of the Foundational Pillars (aka the Forgotten Foundations) as you read through the book!

"There was an idea to bring together a group of remarkable people, to see if we could become something more. So when we needed them, they could fight the battles that we never could."

~ Nick Fury, The Avengers (Marvel Cinematic Universe)

If there's one takeaway from this book, it's that you can't rely on just one pillar or one strategy for lasting well-being. Each pillar is powerful on its own, but together, they form a team of superheroes, protecting us from both the obvious and hidden threats to our health. Incorporating all of them in ways that fit our unique needs and preferences isn't just important—it's essential.

NUTRITION (WHICH INCLUDES HYDRATION!)

Nutrients are what we're made of— they're the fundamental building blocks of our bodies. They provide the energy we need and fuel our intricate physiological processes that sustain life.

ENVIRONMENT—
EMBRACING NATURE, MINIMIZING POLLUTANTS

By connecting with nature, we tap into a powerful resource that supports our health and fosters a sense of peace and balance. Pollutants, which are pervasive, can have serious adverse effects on our health. The goal is to minimize exposure whenever possible and support our bodies in efficiently eliminating the ones we can't avoid.

REGULATION OF THE NERVOUS SYSTEM

This is about discovering our Zen—learning to be the calm amidst the chaos and tapping into our inner strength. The more resilient we become to stress, the happier, more productive, and healthier we become.

FITNESS AND MOVEMENT

Enhancing our strength, agility, endurance, and flow is training for life's biggest challenges—the power to lift and carry, adapt smoothly to sudden changes, move faster and longer, recover from injury or illness, and keep energy and vitality flowing freely through the body.

SLEEP—REST, REPAIR, AND RECHARGE TIME

Restorative sleep and intentional downtime are vital for sustainable health. They're the reset button for our body and mind. Sleep is the body's natural repair mechanism, essential for physical recovery, mental clarity, and emotional balance. Quality rest makes implementing the other pillars that much easier!

And for superhero fans, I've paired each pillar with an Avenger for a fun twist:

NUTRITION (WHICH INCLUDES HYDRATION!)

Captain America

His remarkable strength and vitality stem from the Super-Soldier Serum, which acts like a powerful nutritional boost, enhancing his physical abilities to superhuman levels.

ENVIRONMENT— EMBRACING NATURE, MINIMIZING POLLUTANTS

Black Panther

He draws strength from the natural resources of his homeland, Wakanda, and embodies a deep respect for the environment and its preservation.

Black Widow

She is a master of espionage, skilled at detecting hidden threats and navigating risky environments. (Black widow spiders are also known for their poisonous venom.)

REGULATION OF THE NERVOUS SYSTEM

The Hulk

The key to controlling his rage is self-mastery of his mind and emotions.

FITNESS AND MOVEMENT

Thor

His commanding stature, immense power, and ability to move fluidly in battle exemplify the significance of physical capability.

SLEEP: REST, REPAIR, AND RECHARGE TIME

Iron Man

His genius relies on recharging and upgrading his iconic suit, upgrading it for maximum efficiency.

OUR AUTHOR TEAM

Now here's the most special part of all— this book is a true collaboration!

Healthy for Life has brought together its own group of superheroes. The authors who have joined me are a remarkable group of people—each with their own health expertise, passions, and unique perspectives—to tackle the most important mission of all: helping us guide the kids in our lives toward a healthier, more resilient, and vitality-filled future.

Each author has written a chapter within a designated pillar. Each chapter shares a very personal story and teaches a fundamental health skill. Together, these skills will become tools in your toolbox that you and the children in your care can readily utilize when navigating active health concerns and while taking steps to prevent future ones from happening.

Our authors come from an array of health-related specialties—doctors, a dentist, nutritionists, physical therapists, health coaches, educators, and even health-tech founders. As you read through the book, you'll hear each unique voice and feel each passionate message. You'll get to know the authors a bit, and you'll have easy access to the resources each provides. Our hope is for you to have many "aha" moments and be inspired to continue to learn about whatever resonates most with you.

WHO THIS BOOK IS FOR

This book is for the adults in kids' lives—parents, teachers, mentors, and caregivers—who want to understand essential health concepts, develop key skills to model them and gain the wisdom to guide those in their care. Whether guiding young children, supporting teens, or helping grown kids navigate adulthood, this becomes a win-win for multiple generations.

It's also for anyone, with or without children in their lives, who cares about long-term health and building a strong foundation for a healthy life trajectory.

HOW TO READ THIS BOOK

Healthy for Life is designed to be a practical guide. Our approach is organized around five foundational pillars, each essential for nurturing health and resilience in today's world.

Structure of Each Pillar

At the beginning of each pillar, you'll find a brief overview that introduces the essential concepts related to that topic. These provide a framework from which you can springboard additional learning and exploration.

The unique structure of the book allows you to learn about a few of the concepts within each pillar in a compelling insightful way. Each chapter has a message that the author feels compelled to share far and wide.

You'll read about each author's transformative story, and learn about simple but valuable skills that you can start to implement almost immediately. The skill section includes both the science and concepts, as well actionable steps.

Remember, the pillars are interconnected. The insights from one pillar often complement and enhance those from another. We encourage you to take notes, highlight passages that resonate with you, and share your thoughts with others. This book is a tool for growth and transformation, and your engagement will help unlock its full potential.

Our book's website is www.healthyforlifebook.com. There, you can find resource pages to correlate with each chapter.

Here's to learning, leading, and living well!

CHAPTER 1

BEFORE IT'S TOO LATE

WHAT TRUE PREVENTIVE CARE MEANS

Ilana Zablozki-Amir, MD, DipABPMR, IFMCP

"The time to repair the roof is when the sun is shining."

~ John F. Kennedy

MY STORY

"They found a spot on Daddy's lung."

I was months into my sports medicine fellowship, driving back from providing pre-participation physical exams at a nearby college, when I got the call from my mom. She sounded petrified.

"It'll be fine," I told her, believing it with all my heart. "He has no symptoms, feels great, and even if it is cancer, it was caught early. We'll go through more evaluations, and you'll see, everything will be okay." But we weren't so lucky.

Earlier that day, my father had gone for his routine check-up with his cardiologist, someone he deeply respected. He had no complaints, but given his cardiovascular history, he checked in yearly as advised. As part of his preventive evaluation, they performed a chest x-ray. That's when they found the small spot. It was September 1997.

In October, a lung CT scan revealed two spots—one on each lung. Biopsies confirmed what we feared: both were cancer. A close family friend, also a physician, arranged for my father's case to be discussed at New York University Medical Center's grand rounds. The goal was to understand the relationship between the two spots and determine the best course of action.

I don't recall exactly how they concluded that it was two separate cancers, not one metastatically spread to the other. Nor do I know how the treatment would've changed if they had thought otherwise. I didn't think to ask. Their plan, though aggressive—two surgeries to remove portions of each lung—sounded optimistic. *Why question it?*

I vividly remember sitting in the waiting room during the first surgery. A *People* magazine cover lay beside me, dedicated to one of my favorite singers, John Denver. He had tragically died in a plane crash less than two weeks earlier. Life was feeling surreal.

"The surgery was a success," the surgeon reported, reassuring my mom, brother, and me. He removed the intended lung tissue without complications, and my dad was recovering. After several days in the hospital, my father came home, trying to resume his life, allowing his scar to heal, and managing his pain while waiting for the next surgery.

Despite my optimism, a deep concern settled within me. "We have to give my father a grandchild," I told my husband. It felt urgent. "He needs to have that opportunity in life, it wouldn't be fair if he couldn't experience that joy." We hadn't even considered having a baby anytime soon, as we were both still in the final stages of our professional training. But it suddenly made sense. By God's grace, I got pregnant quickly, and my journey as both a new mother and a daughter fighting for her father's life began.

With an unexpected cough appearing, the second surgery was moved up. I still feel sickened when I recall his post-operative care. One of my most heartbreaking memories is seeing my father—a proud, brilliant, kind, and humble man— pleading silently with his eyes for help, as he suffered from a severe but easily preventable side effect from his pain medication. His smile always warm and full of hope, remained, even in his agony.

His health spiraled downward from there. The spread of the cancer was difficult to control despite ultimately including chemotherapy and radiation. My gosh, the chemotherapy. Yes, it can be lifesaving, but it's simultaneously destructive not just to the cancer but also to the body and the being.

In those days, the pre-Google internet was in its infancy, but still a valuable resource. My brother and I spent most of our waking hours searching for anti-cancer complementary therapies—soups, teas, herbs, enzymes. Their successes were mostly anecdotal but promising! We found names of doctors who incorporated nutritional protocols and off-label treatments. This became even more crucial as my father's nutrition waned during chemo. We compiled our research in a black loose-leaf notebook, desperately grasping for anything that could help.

By March 1998, my father's health deteriorated significantly, but he was still fighting. Then came a pivotal moment for me as a physician. I saw that in the following week, a medical conference was coming to New York, focused on alternative and holistic cancer therapies. It felt like fate— *just what we needed*. I attended, and from the very first lecture, I sat there dumbfounded. They discussed alternative treatments that were showing much success in other countries, the dangers of environmental exposures (like with heavy use of pesticides), and the crucial role of the immune system in the gut. And I learned more there about nutrition than I ever learned in medical school.

I returned home energized, ready to boost my father's nutrition and fly him to Germany for hyperthermia treatments. But we couldn't go until he was stronger. Sadly, his health declined too rapidly. He passed away in April 1998, just seven months after that routine check-up when he felt so well. I was six months pregnant. Three months later, my first son was born, carrying my father's name in his honor.

When my father died, I felt he had been let down by the medical system he trusted. His primary care doctor never addressed the risks that should've been proactively managed. His oncology team, though filled with experts, had no knowledge about any promising complementary therapies. They didn't offer solutions for the side effects of treatment. Other than telling him to "eat ice cream to keep up calories," they overlooked the importance of nutrition as his body battled both the cancer and the toxicity of chemo.

I thought about all the patients I cared for over the years—so many debilitated by chronic conditions—who were also failed by the system. And the many doctors, like me, who were never taught the true possibilities within healthcare. It was disheartening.

I vowed that my father's death wouldn't be in vain. My paradigm shift would be the good that came from his loss, and my tribute to him. Since then, prevention has become the driving force behind everything I do.

Fast forward 26 years, and my understanding of preventive health has evolved through countless hours of education, treating diverse needs of patients, engaging within my community, and my staunch mission to protect the health trajectories of the people I love.

THE SKILL

UNDERSTANDING TRUE PREVENTIVE CARE

As excited as I get when I hear the word *prevention*, I recognize the concept has its challenges. This may be the reason why preventive medicine hasn't been embraced more widely.

First, prevention is often vague. There are countless things to prevent, many actions to implement, and it can be hard to know where to find guidance.

Second, the idea of prevention doesn't always compel action. While its importance is clear, investing time, energy, and money in something that may never pose a problem can feel less valuable.

In our healthcare system, discussions about prevention tend to be shortsighted. Historically, they've centered around vaccines, screening tests for existing diseases (like mammograms and colonoscopies), and public health initiatives. However, as you'll see below, there is much more to consider.

Finally, gauging success can be difficult without objective measures to track progress. I refer to this as the "Prevention Paradox"—if done well, you might question whether those preventive measures were even necessary in the first place.

However, acting before a problem arises is where the greatest impact can be made. Many health conditions—such as heart disease, stroke, certain cancers, diabetes, osteoporosis, dementia, and a range of chronic diseases—are largely preventable. With the right choices and consistent actions, we can significantly reduce the risk of developing these conditions or mitigate their impact on our lives.

Your health—and your child's health—are much more in your control than you may realize. Many people feel disheartened, believing their genes determine their health outcomes, leaving them feeling powerless about their future. This sense of helplessness often leads to a passive mindset, where individuals feel that their efforts won't make a real difference. However, the field of epigenetics shows us that the influence of our genes isn't set in stone. Epigenetic science explores how our environment and choices can affect gene behavior without altering the DNA itself (DNA is what genes are made of). It's now well established that our daily choices, habits, and surroundings significantly influence gene expression.

Think of your genes as a set of instructions for how your body should function. Imagine them as having a light switch: having a gene doesn't mean it's always "on." Your environment—whether it's the food you consume, missing nutrients, the stress you experience, or exposure to toxins—can flip these switches, turning genes "on" or "off." When a gene is activated, it instructs your body to function in a certain way, affecting, among everything else, your immune system, energy levels, mood, how much cholesterol your body retains, and even the way your cells repair themselves. These instructions can set you up for long-lasting health or lead to a spiral of chronic disease.

START EARLY

Diseases like cancer and other chronic conditions often develop quietly over many years—even decades—before symptoms or noticeable tumors appear. Cellular damage can begin long before we're aware of it. There's always some wear and tear occurring, especially as we age, and certain cells may be genetically predisposed. Additionally, factors such as exposure to harmful chemicals, poor nutrition, and stress can exacerbate this damage. By the time a disease surfaces, it has often been progressing unnoticed for a long time. Taking action early gives the body the best chance to defend itself.

Our bodies possess natural defense mechanisms that protect against the repercussions of damaged, dysfunctional cells. From promoting programmed cell death (apoptosis) to repairing DNA, these mechanisms are essential for maintaining health. However, over time, they can become overburdened and depleted.

We can support our natural systems in catching and repairing damage before it leads to more serious issues by maintaining balance—reducing harmful influences when possible and keeping our defenses robust with factors like sound nutrition, fitness, effective communication, a healthy microbiome, and adequate rest. While this may seem overwhelming, it all boils down to implementing foundational habits— what we discuss throughout this book.

IMPLEMENTING A PREVENTIVE ACTION PLAN

To effectively implement a preventive action plan, start by making things concrete:

1. **Articulate What You're Trying to Prevent:** Clearly define your health concerns.

2. **Determine the Urgency of Your Actions:** Assess how immediate your preventive measures need to be.

Prevention can be classified into three categories, or stages. Understanding these stages is helpful when assessing risk and creating goals and strategies for an action plan. A preventive mindset can apply at any stage of health, but the greatest impact occurs when acting as early as possible.

- **Primary Prevention:** Prevent disease or injury before it occurs. At this stage, there is no specific history or detectable findings.

- **Secondary Prevention:** Identify a disease or injury early on, before it has a chance to progress and make a significant impact.

- **Tertiary Prevention:** Prevent recurrence or progression of an existing or previous life-altering illness or injury.

Consider this scenario: You're concerned about heart disease because a relative died in his 50s from a heart attack, and you don't want to follow the same path. You have no symptoms, but your cholesterol is slightly high, and your doctor recently told you that you're fine. Now what? How do you know what your risk at this moment actually is, and how extensive you need to be with your action plan?

Here are some questions to consider:

1. What is the specific concern? *What is my risk of dying from a heart attack?*

2. Is there existing heart disease? *I don't know, but my doctor said I'm fine.*

3. What did your doctor test for? *He did a blood test and checked for everything.*

4. Do you know what he checked specifically? *Other than my cholesterol, which was found to be a little bit high, I don't know. But it seemed to be a lot of tests.*

5. Did he perform any diagnostic evaluations of your heart? *Yeah, he did an EKG and said my heart was fine.*

6. Did he mention checking your blood vessels for plaque that could increase your risk for a heart attack? *Isn't that what the EKG was for?* No, it's not. There are different tests for that. *Oh, I didn't know; I just assumed he did everything necessary.*

I wish I could say this is a fictional scenario, but it isn't. It's a conversation that happens all too often. Regrettably, not asking the right questions can lead to a false sense of security and confusion about what to do next.

In this case, we still don't know which preventive stage you'd fall into. You may be classified in the primary stage since you have no symptoms and have never been diagnosed with heart disease. However, heart disease is often silent until it isn't, making it a leading cause of death worldwide.

Ultimately, if you have the appropriate testing and discover plaque in your arteries, you'll automatically shift to the secondary or tertiary prevention stage. Here, controlling risk factors and diligently implementing strategies to prevent plaque from growing become critical, as your margin for error diminishes. By combining this information with additional heart-related biomarkers on physical examination and blood testing, you can gain a clearer understanding of your risk level, the aggressiveness of treatment needed, and how to monitor it.

PROACTIVE HEALTH

In one of my favorite books, *The Seven Habits of Highly Effective People*, author Stephen Covey outlines key habits for success, starting with "Be Proactive." This habit emphasizes your power to shape your life through choices and mindset. It involves recognizing that you're not just a product of your environment or circumstances and that you have the freedom to choose your response.

Being proactive focuses on what you can control, avoids blaming others, and encourages initiative. It involves planning ahead and making thoughtful decisions based on your values rather than reacting impulsively to emotions or external pressures. This approach requires more effort than simply going along with whatever happens, fostering a more energetic and active mindset.

Proactive health refers to a perspective of prevention that emphasizes actively enhancing and maintaining well-being through positive lifestyle choices and habits. It's the earliest and most robust form of prevention, extending beyond regular check-ups, screenings, and vaccinations.

THE FOUR CORNERSTONES OF A PROACTIVE ACTION PLAN

1. **Prioritize the Pillars:** Proactively and consistently implement strategies within all five Healthy for Life Pillars (NERFS). These foundations impact everything and can be considered "pro-actions."

2. **Recognize Your Risks:** Identify your unique risks for particular health concerns. Consider your family history, past or current environmental exposures, traumatic events you may have experienced, potential nutritional deficiencies, and awareness of red-flag symptoms. There are now readily available tests that can help you understand your unique genetic needs.

3. **Understand Your Terrain:** Utilize diagnostic testing to assess what's happening inside your body. This can include a combination of physical examinations, blood tests, imaging tests, and physiological assessments that provide feedback about your current health.

4. **Build Your Toolbox and Team:** Continuously expand your skill set, resources, knowledge of effective therapies, and support network to protect and restore your health.

All four are crucial. Taking one type of action without considering the others can lead to incomplete plans. You may lead a very healthy lifestyle, but you also need to understand how it impacts your health terrain and whether it's making a difference.

THE PARADOX OF EARLY DETECTION

Early detection saves lives! It means identifying issues like cancerous growths or artery blockages in the heart while they are still small. However, as in my father's case, finding a condition at this stage may be too late.

Prevention must begin with early action and a thorough understanding of your health landscape. Are there signs of inflammation, oxidative stress, nutrient deficiencies, blood sugar imbalances, immune dysfunction, impaired hormone communication, or other markers of a dysfunctional physiology? Are your body's defenses and offenses working as they should?

In hindsight, even though lung cancer wasn't on our radar, I would've ensured my father understood the importance of a foundational, balanced lifestyle. I would've considered his overall health risks, recognizing how they primed him for cancer growth: his history of cardiovascular events, past smoking, a challenging diet, and work-related asbestos exposure. Additionally, the trauma he experienced as a teenager in the Soviet Union during World War II—losing his entire family to execution in a city square near Minsk—might have had lasting impacts, especially on his lung health. I've learned that the energetic signature of grief tends to be associated with the lungs.

I would've tracked his health with comprehensive testing for red-flag physiological dysfunctions—examining what was happening "upstream" before any disease developed. And I would've equipped him with a toolkit with a wide variety of resources to complement or preclude the need for medications or surgery if and when any health issues arose.

ACTIVITY:

Overflowing Bucket Prevention Exercise

Goal:

The goal is to identify what fills and drains your health "bucket". This is a simple and powerful first next step that you, the children in your care, and most anyone can do, towards being proactive with self-care.

Materials:

Sheet of Paper; Markers; Sticky Notes or Index Cards

Instructions:

1. **Draw Your Bucket:** On the paper, draw a large bucket to represent your overall health.

2. **Identify Drains:** Reflect on things that drain your energy or negatively impact your health (e.g., stressors, unhealthy habits, toxic relationships). Write down each drain on a sticky note or card and place them outside of the bucket, representing holes or leaks.

3. **Identify Fills:** Think about activities, habits, and people that fill your bucket (e.g., exercise, hobbies, time with loved ones, self-care practices) Write these on sticky notes and place them inside the bucket.

4. **Visualize Balance:** Are there more drains than fills? Consider how the "holes" can be mitigated by adding more "fills".

5. **Create an Action Plan:** Choose one to three actions to take over the next week to either reduce drains or increase fills. Write these actions down and place them around your bucket for motivation.

6. **Reflect:** After a week, review your bucket and notice any changes in your mood or energy.

I believe that once we embrace proactive prevention as individuals, the healthcare system as a whole will have no choice but to follow suit. It may take a while, but it's in our hands.

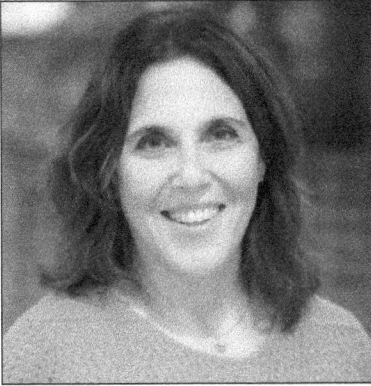

Dr. Ilana Zablozki-Amir is a physician who is a visionary in holistic health and a champion for proactive wellness.

She is board certified in the fields of Physical Medicine and Rehabilitation and Integrative-Holistic Medicine, fellowship-trained in Sports and Musculoskeletal Medicine, a certified practitioner by the Institute for Functional Medicine, and a Precision Nutrition level 2 certified health coach.

Dr. Ilana loves to learn and collaborate! She has pursued extensive continuing education across a wide array of health fields, delving deeply into each foundational health pillar. Her expertise is truly integrative —with an understanding from her experience in allopathic, more conventional medicine, and from more upstream root cause and alternative perspectives.

She is a firm believer that every person is unique, drawing inspiration from works like *Fire Child, Water Child,* and finds joy in uncovering the stories that shape each individual. She tailors her approaches to resonate with each individual's needs and aspirations.

Dr. Ilana is a passionate advocate for a shift in medical paradigms—from predominantly medication-focused healthcare to a model where prevention, early action, root cause understanding, natural healing options, and self-care play an integral role.

As a mother of three boys, now young men, she understands the critical roles that family and community dynamics play in helping to nurture children's understanding and habits of health and well-being.

In her medical practice, she helps people "Understand to Prevent" and designs proactive roadmaps for people of all ages to help navigate their health trajectories. Her target focus is on early action because that's most often when the greatest difference can be made.

Connect with Dr. Ilana:

Websites:
www.brooklynintegrativemedicine.com (www.brooklynim.com)
www.healthyforlifebook.com
Instagram: www.instagram.com/dr.ilanaza   @dr.ilanaza

Dr. Ilana's Hashtags:
#OpenMindsSaveLives
#LookUpstream
#TodayIsTomorrowsUpstream
#PerspectiveIsEverything
#HealthyForLife

PILLAR 1

NUTRITION

You are what you eat, literally.

NUTRITION: AN OVERVIEW

Food is not only our fuel, it's what our cells are made of. It's also a language, with information that speaks directly to our bodies, influencing how our genes express themselves, how our brain functions, and how our cells repair and renew. At the same time, it fosters connection in building relationships, expressing care, and celebrating culture, which in turn enhances well-being.

Food is a central focus in our lives, yet it's so misunderstood. It can be the greatest medicine or a strong health saboteur. Nutrition has lots of nuances. The key is to find within each principle, what works best for you.

Nutrition is such a broad and essential topic that it could fill an encyclopedia, but let's begin with a simple overview of how to think about it. You can use this framework when learning further and as a go-to guide when making daily choices. Please remember that proper foundational nutrition takes lots into consideration. The chapters to come will touch on many of these concepts.

Food:

- Calorie awareness–Not too few, not too many for your goals and needs.
- Macronutrients–Protein, fat, carbohydrate, fiber.
- Micronutrients–Vitamins, minerals.
- Phytonutrients–Powerful, colorful plant compounds.
- Quality–Least processed, least problematic ingredients, not overcooked.
- Diversity–Goal of eating a variety of foods; for example many different types of fruits/veggies in a week.
- Timing–Avoid sugar swings/insulin spikes, finish well before bed.
- Digestion–Chew! and eat in a relaxed state (rest and digest mode).

- Absorption–Ensuring that your intestinal health is supportive of getting what you eat into the body. It's not only what you eat, it's what you absorb!
- Baggage–What else are you getting along with your food—pesticides, teflon, plastic particles, chemicals, hormones, bacteria? Take care to be mindful where and how your food is grown, cooked, stored, handled.
- Troublesome ingredient–Could it be that something is causing an allergy or sensitivity?
- Nuances–Understanding and remembering that what is good for one person, is not necessarily good for another.

Hydration:
- Water! In the form of water, tea, soup, smoothies, fresh produce, and other supportive foods.
- Added boosts of electrolytes/minerals.
- Filtered/purified (because, like food, it also can come with "baggage").
- Goal of approximately how many ounces the body needs per day:

  50% of body weight in pounds (Example: A 160-pound person ideally needs around 80 ounces per day)- may need additional if sweating or other health condition.

Supplements * – Supplemental to food:
- Understand and support your unique needs based on the type of diet you eat, health conditions, functional goals, etc. ie vitamins, minerals, essential fatty acids, essential amino acids; anti-inflammatory, antioxidant, and immune-boosting compounds; blood flow support; microbiome support, etc.
- *It's rare to be able to get all you need from food. Most of us don't have enough variety in our diet or food that has fully retained its quality.

CHAPTER 2

THE HEART OF NUTRITION

PREVENTING HEART DISEASE THROUGHOUT YOUR LIFE

Giovanni Campanile, MD, FACC

"Do the best you can until you know better. Then, when you know better, do better."

~ Maya Angelou

MY STORY

I completed my Interventional Cardiology Fellowship at New England Deaconess Hospital in Boston. I was on-call for the emergency room of a New England hospital for the first time out of training. It was a Sunday, and I was home with my wife and two children. My beeper went off (yes, beeper—I didn't have a cell phone), and it was the emergency room calling me about a patient who was en route and experienced a cardiac arrest. I jumped into my car and drove as fast as possible to the hospital. When I got there, the EMTs were rolling the patient, Peter, into the Critical Care room of the emergency department. The paramedics and the patient's wife gave me a brief history of events.

Peter was mowing the lawn and collapsed in front of his wife and daughter. Peter's wife was a nurse and felt that he didn't have a pulse and initiated CPR immediately while the daughter called 911. Peter's wife continued CPR until the paramedics arrived. The paramedics assessed the situation very quickly, continued CPR, and connected Peter to an automatic external defibrillator (AED), which shocked Peter multiple times during his transport to the hospital.

When I first examined Peter, I noticed things didn't look good—he had no pulse. I looked at his heart with an ultrasound machine, which revealed no heart movement whatsoever. So, we continued CPR, placed a breathing tube into his trachea, and gave him intravenous medications to jump-start his heart.

I spoke to Peter's wife and explained that the prognosis did not look good. She responded: "Please do everything you can to save him."

At this point, I activated the cardiac catheterization laboratory (cath lab). Within minutes, I looked into his heart arteries to find he was experiencing a heart attack with complete occlusion of the "widow maker" coronary artery in the front of his heart. Three coronary arteries feed the heart muscle: the left anterior descending (LAD), the left circumflex (LCX), and the right coronary artery (RCA). The artery that was blocked in Peter's case was the LAD.

Within 15 minutes of Peter's arrival at the cath lab, I opened the blockage, which re-established blood flow to a large part of Peter's heart. I then placed a metal scaffold called a stent to ensure that the artery remained open.

Peter's heart then started to beat on its own, his blood pressure stabilized, and he was transferred to the Coronary Care Unit for further observation and treatment.

I spoke to his wife immediately after the procedure. "The stent placement was a success. We restored blood flow, and the heart is now beating normally." However, Peter was still unconscious, and we didn't know if he had brain damage. We performed a CT scan of the head, which didn't show evidence of a stroke. However, a CT scan cannot always determine if there has been permanent brain damage.

So, for around 12 hours, we weren't sure if Peter would make a neurological recovery. However, around that time, Peter woke up. From that point on, he made a remarkable recovery. He could breathe independently and was taken off the ventilator. Less than a week later, he was discharged, walking on his own with average mental capacity.

I followed Peter very carefully after that, making sure he did everything possible to prevent this from ever happening again. On one of his visits, he asked, "Why did this happen to me?"

The simple answer to Peter's question was that a blood clot developed in a heart artery and stopped blood flow to a significant part of his heart. The more complicated part of the answer is why a blockage was created in the first place.

Since I treated Peter, I've treated thousands of other patients with heart attacks, coronary blockages, and a myriad of heart ailments. Somewhere in my career, I, too, asked the same question Peter asked me all those years ago. Why does this happen to so many people in the Western world, and what should we do to prevent this epidemic?

This led me to change my perspective and approach to my practice completely.

Around this time, I had the good fortune of meeting Dr. Joseph Pizzorno, who was the President of Bastyr University in Washington State (one of the most highly regarded schools of naturopathic medicine). He introduced me to naturopathic medicine. This was a watershed moment for me—it opened my eyes to the idea that we must take a holistic approach to the patient to heal. This was quite different from what we learned in traditional medical training.

Since then, I spent many hours learning as much as I could about naturopathic, integrative, and functional medicine. I have also become educated in nutrition. I became the Director of the Dean Ornish Reversal of Heart Disease program for Atlantic Health, where I witnessed firsthand that lifestyle change was mighty and could reverse established coronary artery disease.

IN ORDER TO PREVENT A HEART ATTACK IN AN ADULT, PREVENTION STARTS DURING PREGNANCY AND CONTINUES LIFELONG

We now know that coronary disease can begin before birth, influenced by the mother's diet and cholesterol levels, which directly affect the developing fetus. We also know that coronary artery disease is almost 100% secondary to lifestyle choices, such as poor diet, lack of exercise, obesity, stress, and inadequate sleep.

As in Peter's case, these factors accumulate during childhood, adolescence, and adulthood, leading to conditions that can cause heart attacks.

Autopsy studies from motor vehicle accidents and wartime casualties have shown that nearly every American under age 20 already has fatty streaks in their coronary arteries—early signs of atherosclerotic plaque–which is the cause of hardening and blockages of arteries. These plaques continue to progress through the years, culminating in heart attacks in people in their 50s and 60s. In contrast, similar autopsy studies on people in non-western countries with very different lifestyles and diets show almost no coronary disease, signifying that this is an entirely preventable lifestyle disease.

Studies of modern-day foragers, such as the Tsimane in Bolivia and the Hadza in Tanzania, reveal that they tend to have lower blood pressure, naturally low cholesterol levels, and almost no coronary artery disease. These groups naturally incorporate physical activity into their daily lives. The Hadza, for instance, walk 8-12 kilometers each day, climb trees, and dig for root vegetables. Their diet is made up primarily of whole, unprocessed foods, including many plants, fibers, nuts, seeds, meat, fish, and occasional honey. They consume lean meat from wild animals, free from hormones and chemicals, and avoid added sugars, fats, and salt—common staples in modern Western diets.

To help prevent heart disease in children, they should never be exposed to tobacco or smoke, maintain a healthy body weight, engage in at least 60 minutes of daily moderate or vigorous exercise, limit sedentary time (TV, computers, cell phones, gaming), and eat a diet rich in colorful plant-based foods with very limited ultra-processed foods (excessive in added sugars, fats, or salt). They should also maintain cholesterol under 170 milligrams/deciliter (mg/dL), normal blood pressure, and fasting blood sugar below

100 mg/dL. A child who follows these healthful habits can add an estimated 12 years to their lifespan—a fantastic gift!

The cornerstone of all these lifestyle factors is diet. Unfortunately, 70% of the calories in most American children today come from ultra-processed foods (UPF), which are linked to higher body weight, higher blood sugar levels, higher cholesterol, lower cardiovascular fitness, and higher rates of diabetes and cancer. In addition, children accustomed to eating UPFs develop an aversion to healthy plant food and prefer soft, sweet, artificially flavored foods.

UNDERSTAND THAT WE ARE ALL PART OF THE ECOSYSTEM THAT SURROUNDS US

We are all part of a vast ecosystem, both inside and out. The microbiome, made up of bacteria, viruses, and fungi, lives in and on our bodies. Evolving with us over millions of years, these "friendly" microbes protect us from harmful bugs and produce substances that help us thrive. Together, we form a symbiotic relationship: we provide a habitat, and in return, these "friendly" microbes protect us from harmful invaders and produce beneficial substances that support our health.

Our microbiome is so extensive that the number of microbial cells in our bodies matches our human cells. This raises an intriguing question: who is the true "host"—us or them? In fact, we are just one part of an intricate ecosystem that includes not only the microbes within us but also the earth, plants, water, and all living systems around us. This interconnectedness suggests that caring for every part of our environment impacts our own health and the health of the larger community.

The journey of a healthy microbiome begins at birth. A newborn acquires its first microbes through the mother's birth canal, skin, and even feces. Breast milk and skin-to-skin contact further support this early microbiome development. This natural closeness between mothers and infants may have evolved, in part, to help create an ideal microbial environment, benefiting both mother and child. By age three, a child's microbiome typically resembles that of an adult.

The health of our microbiome has ripple effects that reach our hearts. Just as the heart circulates blood to nourish every part of our body, the microbiome regulates processes that protect and sustain the heart. This connection highlights the broader theme that our bodies are highly interconnected systems—what affects one area, like the gut, can profoundly impact another, like the heart. A well-nourished microbiome plays a key role in keeping our heart healthy. Whole real food, rich in fiber and nutrients, does this.

HEALTH SPAN

We don't want to live longer just for the sake of living longer. What we all want for ourselves and our children is an improved *health span*, which means the length of time a person is healthy, not just alive. A corollary of the health span concept is referred to as *contraction of morbidity*, which is the goal of decreasing the period of chronic illness in one's life to a shorter time frame. In other words, to push the age at which a person first experiences a chronic disease as far into the future as possible. Centenarians and super-centenarians (110+ years of age) die of the same chronic illnesses as the rest of the population; however, they suffer these illnesses at a much later time of their lives and for a significantly shorter period. So, by directing your children onto a path of optimal wellness, you'll be giving them a gift that will help them throughout childhood and adolescence and far later in their lives when they become adults and elderly. This is why it has been shown that the influence of an optimal lifestyle is passed down through many generations, not only because the knowledge is passed down but also because of epigenetics—the actual genetic improvements are also passed down.

THE SKILL

PREVENTIVE CARDIOLOGY: HOW TO BETTER ASSESS YOUR PERSONALIZED HEART ATTACK RISK

Heart attacks are something everyone wants to prevent. The earlier we intervene, the better. While we've discussed the importance of proactive health for children, it's equally vital for adults, especially those with past health concerns or a risk-inducing lifestyle history. Peter's story was a powerful reminder of how suddenly a heart attack can strike and the devastation it can leave behind.

THE URGENCY OF CARDIOVASCULAR HEALTH

Every **1.7 seconds**, someone dies from cardiovascular disease. Shockingly, over **50% of heart attack victims** experience no prior symptoms, and **75% of artery blockages** that cause heart attacks are often missed by standard tests. This means millions of heart attacks could theoretically be prevented with better risk assessment and early intervention.

A heart attack occurs when blood flow to a part of the heart is blocked, causing oxygen deprivation and muscle damage. This is often caused by plaque buildup in the arteries. To prevent this, stabilizing and reversing plaque is essential.

ASSESSING YOUR RISK

Your doctor should review risk factors and warning signs of poor artery health. A list of these, and more information about the tests below can be found on the chapter resource webpage. Online calculators like the ASCVD Risk Estimator here...

https://tools.acc.org/ascvd-risk-estimator-plus/#!/calculate/estimate/

...provide a starting point, but remember—they don't account for everything, such as family history or environmental factors. Even low-risk scores warrant attention and regular check-ins with your healthcare provider.

ADVANCED DIAGNOSTIC STUDIES

1. Blood Testing

Traditional tests that check "good" more protective HDL and so-called "bad" more risky LDL cholesterol may be limited in their ability to predict heart attack risk. Newer and more thorough assessments focus on:

- **Cholesterol particle quality and size** and the number of LDL particles.
- **Apolipoproteins (ex.ApoB)**—a better predictor of cardiovascular risk than LDL.

- **Lipoprotein(a) / Lp(a)**, a genetic marker linked to heart disease, with new therapies emerging to lower its levels.
- **Artery Inflammation Markers** can indicate underlying arterial health concerns.

Some panels even analyze cholesterol origins—either from liver production or gut absorption, offering insights to guide treatment.

2. Imaging to Peek Inside the Arteries

Modern imaging technologies provide clear visuals of artery health.

- **CT Coronary Calcium Score:** This noninvasive test measures calcium in the coronary arteries. Scores range from 0 (low risk) to over 300 (high risk).
- **Coronary CT Angiography (CCTA):** This test uses IV contrast for 3D images, identifying both calcified and non-calcified plaques, the latter being more dangerous as it's more likely to cause heart attacks. Using AI, CCTA can distinguish between inflamed and stable plaque, enhancing personalized diagnosis and treatment.

THE RISKS OF RELYING ON STRESS TESTS ALONE

Stress tests often detect coronary artery disease only in advanced stages, potentially providing a false sense of security. Advanced imaging, like CCTA with AI, offers earlier, clearer insights, making it easier to catch issues before they progress and monitor improvements.

Taking a proactive approach to heart health means leveraging today's advanced tools to understand and reduce your unique risk of heart disease.

LIVE WELL DELICIOUSLY

There are many things we can do to prevent, halt, and even reverse plaque buildup in the arteries. One of the most critical and best first lifestyle steps is diet.

The Mediterranean diet is widely considered one of the healthiest eating patterns in the world, which has been shown to improve heart health, reduce inflammation, and support weight management.

By focusing on wholesome, unprocessed foods, this diet not only helps prevent chronic diseases such as heart disease, diabetes, and cancer, but it also promotes longevity, with studies linking it to a longer, healthier life.

PRINCIPLES OF A MEDITERRANEAN DIET:

- Local, Seasonal Produce: Fresh vegetables and fruits are central, chosen based on what's in season to ensure peak flavor and nutrient density.

- Olive Oil as a Daily Staple: Extra virgin olive oil, rich in antioxidants, healthy fats, polyphenols and vitamins is used generously for cooking and dressing.

- Lean Proteins: Seafood, along with legumes (chickpeas, lentils) provides protein and omega-3s. The best fish for omega-3 content are the SMASH fish (salmon, mackerel, anchovies, sardines and herring).

- Whole Grains and Ancient Breads: Traditional Sicilian breads made from whole grains or ancient grains are a dietary mainstay that can support gut health. These grains are rich in nutrients and contain all parts of the grain—bran, germ, and endosperm—each contributing unique health benefits. You may find conflicting information about grains, as some people may need to avoid them due to digestive issues or sensitivities. You may also find that different cooking methods help with digestibility.

- Minimal Processed Foods and Red Meat: Processed items are rare, and red meat is eaten sparingly, focusing instead on plant-based and seafood-based meals.

- Herbs and Simple Flavors: Fresh herbs like oregano, rosemary, and basil enhance flavor and health benefits without added sauces.

- Fruit for Dessert: Instead of sugary desserts, seasonal fruits are enjoyed, making the diet naturally low in added sugars.

My wife, Sandra Cammarata (also a *Healthy for Life* author), and I designed *The Sicilian Secret Diet* to blend Mediterranean eating with the rich, traditional flavors of Sicily. Our motto, *Live Well Deliciously*, highlights our belief that a healthy diet should be as enjoyable as it is nourishing.

Sicilian cuisine—a unique mix of Roman, Greek, Arab, Spanish, French, and Jewish influences—embodies balanced, flavorful, and mindful eating as a way to lasting wellness. And when enjoying in a social setting, it becomes a sustainable and empowering lifestyle for overall well-being.

"If we could give every individual the right amount of nourishment and exercise, not too little and not too much, we would have found the safest way to health."

~ Hippocrates (450 BC)

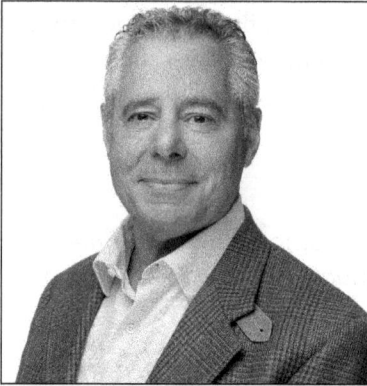

Dr. Giovanni Campanile is a Harvard-trained cardiologist. He is the former director of the Dean Ornish Intensive Cardiac Rehabilitation Program and of Integrative Nutrition and Integrative Cardiology at the Chambers Center for Well Being. He is quadruple board certified in Internal Medicine, Cardiology, Interventional Cardiology, and the American Board of Integrative and Holistic Medicine. He is an Assistant Professor of Medicine at Rutgers New Jersey Medical School and has been an instructor for doctors specializing in cardiology at Lenox Hill Hospital in New York City and Columbia University Mount Sinai, Miami.

Dr. Campanile was a researcher at the world-renowned Framingham Heart Study and has investigated integrative modalities with the National Institute of Health, Rutgers New Jersey Medical School, Duke University, and Yale University.

He was a cardiologist for former President of the United States, George H.W. Bush, and is a contributing editor and medical writer for Shape and Men's Fitness Magazines.

Dr. Campanile has been practicing Integrative Cardiology for over 15 years and has been a member of an advisory board at Bastyr University. He has been an instructor of Nutrition, Herbology, and Integrative Medicine at Florida Atlantic University and is a certified aromatherapist. He has been named "Top Doctor" in cardiology by New Jersey Monthly Magazine for multiple years.

He and his wife Sandra Cammarata, who is also a physician, have written the popular book, *The Sicilian Secret Diet Plan*, which is a book on the Mediterranean Diet from Sicily. They have a well-followed podcast, The Sicilian Secret Diet, where they interview recognized personalities and authors in the world of wellness medicine. They are currently working on a follow-up book and film in Sicily.

Together they've formulated a Mediterranean Diet supplement (available on Amazon), *Healthy to 100*, which contains all of the key nutritional components of the Mediterranean Diet in a convenient formulation.

Connect with Dr. Campanile:

Websites:

https://functionalheart.com

https://siciliansecret.com

https://coraeon.com

Instagram: @siciliansecretdiet

Office phone for appointments: (908)936-1652

CHAPTER 3

HOW TO BE CONFIDENT AND CREATIVE IN THE KITCHEN

PREPARING NOURISHING MEALS THAT HEAL

Monique Bogni, CNC, CHHC

MY STORY

The first time I realized carob wasn't chocolate, I cried. I think I was in second grade when I finally defied my parents' warnings not to share food at school. I remember feeling guilty and scared I'd get into trouble as I reluctantly took a piece of a brownie my friend was innocently offering me.

It looked a lot different than the brownies my mom made. They were darker in color, had a crunchy top, and had a soft middle. I later learned these were made from Betty Crocker Brownie Mix in the classic red box.

I took a tiny bite, and my tastebuds exploded! In one instant, a flood of memories rushed into my mind as I attempted to make sense of what was happening in my mouth: The hot chocolate warming up on the stove with foamy homemade soy milk and being excited to add the amount of honey I wanted; going to the natural food store and getting to pick out my favorite "candy bar," the one with the chewy raisins covered in "chocolate" that felt like a special treat; batch after batch of those soft cakey brownies nesting on the counter, hidden under tin foil on a paper plate, that we all secretly ate throughout the day.

The epiphany came. *Carob is **not** chocolate.* My parents used the words *carob* and *chocolate* interchangeably, and up until that moment, I thought they were the same thing. Although carob and cacao, which chocolate is made from, both come from pods on trees, contain antioxidants, and are used in the same way, they have very distinct flavors.

That afternoon I arrived home from school to find my mom in the kitchen. I yelled, "Carob is not chocolate! You lied to me!" Taken by surprise, she calmly explained that she used carob whenever a recipe called for chocolate because she felt it was healthier. Chocolate contains caffeine, one of the ingredients that made soda off-limits, and carob was caffeine-free. I don't know why I was so surprised to learn this secret. I knew we ate differently than other families. My parents would say they were ahead of their time when it came to healthy eating. They bought everything organic, and I remember shopping at Bread of Life when I was little before it got bought out by Whole Foods.

I remember getting dropped off at birthday parties and cringing as my mom handed over the nitrate-free turkey dogs and *carob* brownies sweetened with honey. At least the diabetic kid felt less awkward because he wasn't allowed to eat the party food either. The irony is that I liked the food my mom prepared for me. And when I sneaked a bite of the bright red and blue frosting from the grocery store cake, I thought it tasted weird and was way too sweet. I knew what unprocessed, whole foods tasted like because that's mostly what my parents made at home. Most everything was made from scratch, even the waffles. Sure, we had cereal, too, but it was boring, unsweetened shredded wheat. Occasionally, I got a glimpse into the forbidden food world. I spent the night at a friend's house, and for breakfast, was served an Eggo waffle hot out of the toaster. They topped it with *I can't believe it's not Butter* and a strange tasting pancake syrup—quite different from real butter and the 100% pure maple syrup I was used to eating.

There were always fruits and vegetables around; we even had an enormous boysenberry bush in the backyard and a lush garden filled with organic produce. In kindergarten, I recall eating a pomegranate at recess, my favorite fruit at the time. A kid came up to me, made a sour face, and asked, "What's that?" I didn't know how to pronounce the name and said,

"I don't know," as I shrugged off that uncomfortable feeling I got when it felt like someone was judging what I ate.

When it came to vegetables, Dad had a talent for making them taste good. As an appetizer, he served up a hot plate of roasted cauliflower drizzled with Newman's Italian dressing with a sprinkling of Parmesan and pepper. Every week my parents picked up fresh tofu made from organic soybeans, long before soy crops became GMO, and pressed out the liquid between two giant wooden blocks. Dad made braised tofu in a cast iron skillet with soy sauce, dried onion flakes, and ketchup and served it alongside sautéed broccoli. It was one of my favorite childhood dishes! Then there was the sautéed chard—I have no idea what sorcery he used to make it taste so buttery (probably lots of butter), but I decided it was the tastiest green from our garden! I particularly liked the chard that had pink and red stems, as these were my favorite colors. It made sense that it was called rainbow chard.

As I got older, sneaking tastes of chips and cookies in those brightly colored snack-sized bags with shiny foil on the inside became a thrilling adventure. My favorites were peanut M&M's and ranch-flavored Doritos. My parents never bought these, of course. However, friends felt bad and thought they were doing me a favor by offering an array of forbidden snacks and candy at recess or when I went over to their house to play.

My parents got divorced when I entered my teen years, and there was far less monitoring of what I ate. I remember the first time I went into a 7-Eleven and had my own money. I hit the Slurpee machine and put every single pink, blue, purple, and Coke flavor into one super-sized paper cup. The fun straw with the scoop on the end was a bonus. I stood in the candy aisle, unable to choose what I wanted. *I knew I liked chocolate, ha!* The details of my junk food habits don't matter, as you get the idea. I had more freedom in high school to eat forbidden foods such as candy, soda, fast food, and everything in between.

I headed into college and experienced much more than the freshman fifteen (a term used to describe the average amount of weight college students gain during their first year). Just before my senior year, I lost my older brother in a car accident. We were very close, and he was much more than a brother to me—he was my mentor, my rock, and one of my best friends. I developed some unhelpful coping strategies that included binging on alcohol and eating takeout food. I remember looking at a giant plate of nachos and deciding I would eat whatever I wanted until I felt numb. Although I didn't know it at the time, I sedated myself with unhealthy, processed food. Weighed down by grief, I didn't care that overeating made me feel physically uncomfortable and sometimes sick. This, of course, led to my weight gain and health issues.

After college, I got a job with a catering company and often ate the decadent food they generously served to staff. One day, while getting ready for work, I struggled to zip up my pants and thought, *I just bought bigger pants. There's no way I'm going up another size! That's it. I have to do something about this.*

I decided to go back to my roots; I began shopping organic and read every nutrition and diet book I could get my hands on. I read the ingredient label on everything packaged and put back anything with chemical additives, as Mom taught me to do early on. I brought in fruits and vegetables in a variety of colors and included as many of these in my diet as I could. I became more mindful about what I put into my body, and I noticed how food made me feel. I had once thought it was normal to feel tired and bloated after meals. By preparing most of my food at home and eating less out of packages, the weight melted off; I healed my chronic constipation and chronic fatigue and eliminated the back pain I thought was a normal part of growing older.

Choosing organic continues to be an important practice to reduce my toxic exposure. Organic means food is produced using natural and sustainable farming practices without most conventional pesticides, herbicides, synthetic fertilizers, and genetically modified components. Meat, poultry, and dairy products come from animals that haven't been given antibiotics or growth hormones or feed contaminated by the chemicals mentioned above, toxins linked to a wide range of health issues. The toxic chemicals sprayed on produce and injected into animals are deemed safe for consumption in small quantities. But that's with limited exposure. We're exposed to toxins daily from multiple sources. It's well known that over time, a cumulative effect can occur with higher doses and can contribute to a host of health concerns.

I once was stopped by someone in the produce aisle as I gathered my items from the organic section. They said, "I apologize for interrupting you, but can you tell me if it's really that important to get organic produce versus nonorganic produce?" I thought for a moment and told them, "The fact that you're in the produce section is what matters, and it's important to start where it feels good to you." In my experience, including more fruits and vegetables and choosing organic whenever possible leads to optimal health.

THE SKILL

I consider fruits and vegetables superfoods because they contain an abundance of immune-boosting antioxidants, vitamins, and minerals. They are the best form of fiber for keeping the digestive tract in working order. As this roughage moves through the intestines, it has a sweeping effect and scrubs out toxins and food waste that get stuck in the pipes throughout your life. They are the clean-up crew and will keep you pooping. Maintaining a healthy gut can have a positive impact on your emotional and mental well-being, prevent disease, give you more energy, and help you sustain a healthy weight.

So, how do you get more fruit and vegetable fiber into your diet from breakfast through dinner? I'm going to share the following easy-to-incorporate strategies:

1. Make vegetables the star of your plate.

2. Eat your leafy greens.

3. Eat the rainbow.

STRATEGY 1: MAKE VEGETABLES THE STAR OF YOUR PLATE

Historically, meat has been the star of the plate, paired with an unexciting vegetable garnish. Instead, make vegetables the star of the show and give other foods a supporting role. Regardless of what you enjoy eating, start focusing on adding more vegetables and leafy greens, then sprinkle in the rest.

Even if you aren't ready to give up some of your favorite inflammatory foods, you can still add in more vegetables. Whether it feels good to eat them raw, peeled, roasted, steamed, blended, or baked, the more you get in, the more satisfied and nourished you will feel throughout your day.

Here is what your plate might look like when you make vegetables the star of your meal:

- Fill two-thirds of your plate with broccoli, asparagus, and arugula, totaling two to four cups of vegetables. The other one-third is filled with organic, grass-fed meat or plant-based protein. If you desire starch, I like to add cooked sweet potatoes and winter squash like pumpkin.

- For a plant-based meal, fill your plate 60-70% with vegetables and leafy greens and the other 30-40% with plant-based protein and complex carbs such as lentils and sweet potatoes or peas and quinoa.

- If you have compromised digestion, eating cooked vegetables can be soothing to the gut. Steaming and boiling are the most hydrating methods for cooking vegetables and are gentler on irritated intestinal walls as they move through. If you're concerned that cooking vegetables reduces their nutrient content, keep in mind you will be ingesting more nutrients by cooking them as opposed to not eating any at all.

- Add some avocado, olives, nuts, or seeds to make your meal more satisfying and interesting.

- Don't forget about fresh and dried fruit to balance flavors. Apples, mandarins, grapes, raisins, and dates offer nice textures and sweetness to savory dishes.

- Sprinkle on some high-quality organic cheese if that's what it's going to take for you to eat a salad or a plate full of vegetables as your main meal. *That's how Dad originally got me to eat them!* In my experience, goat and sheep dairy tend to be easier to digest than cow dairy.

STRATEGY 2: EAT YOUR LEAFY GREENS

Leafy greens are filled with bio-available vitamins and protein. They're one of the most nutrient-dense vegetables we can consume, yet people often undervalue their importance. Or they tend to think the only way to consume them is in a salad. Even then, the greens are not usually the star of the show.

I'm here to shift this mentality and help you get more leafy greens wherever you can!

- Using a measuring cup, put four to eight cups of loosely packed leafy greens such as spinach, kale, butter lettuce, romaine, arugula, green or red leaf lettuce, spring mix, etc., and place your green of choice in a bowl. This can now be the base of any meal. You will be surprised at how filling eating this many leafy greens can be!

- I find that spinach is one of the mildest greens, and you can put a few handfuls into your smoothie, a soup as it finishes cooking, a stir fry, or into cooked grains.

- A great trick is to thinly slice your greens so they are easier to chew and disappear more easily into your dish.

- Green up that simple meal of pasta, stew, or rice and beans! Add four to eight cups of greens like chard, spinach, arugula, kale, etc., when your dish is finished cooking. Stir until they're wilted and incorporated.

- Find it challenging to eat salad, sauté it on the stove to gently cook the ingredients and warm it up.

If you have concerns about oxalates, consider cutting back on higher-oxalate varieties like spinach and opting to cook them, as cooking helps reduce oxalate levels. If you take certain medications like blood thinners, you can speak to your doctor about how best to incorporate them.

STRATEGY 3: EAT THE RAINBOW

Eating a rainbow of fruits and vegetables is essential for optimal health. The diverse range of fibers, antioxidants, and prebiotics found in these foods nourishes the beneficial bacteria in your gut, promoting optimal digestion, boosting immunity, and reducing inflammation. By incorporating a variety of colors into your diet, you can cultivate a thriving gut microbiome, leading to improved overall health and well-being. A colorful plate is a healthy plate!

Here are my favorite strategies for eating the rainbow:

- When shopping at the store, pick one new fruit and vegetable to try each week.

- If you typically buy green apples or green grapes, try picking a different colored apple or grape. If you always buy red bell peppers, try orange or yellow, for example.

- Drink smoothies. Blending fruits and vegetables makes them pre-digested and is a great way to load up on nutrients while being gentle on a sensitive digestive system. Adding spices like cinnamon, ginger, and cayenne can create a warming effect that can also make a smoothie more digestible for some people.

  - How to make a *filling* smoothie: Measure out four to five cups of fruit. Bananas, mango, coconut, avocado, and papaya will add creaminess. You can add a few handfuls of greens for added nutrition. If you need to eat less fruit for health concerns, add frozen chopped zucchini with berries. Blend with one to two cups of filtered water or coconut water. Add a little raw honey or a few pitted dates for more sweetness if desired. Add avocado, flax, chia, pumpkin seeds, or coconut yogurt for some healthy fat.

- If it doesn't feel good to eat raw fruit, bake a fruit crisp. Apples and berries are my favorite combination.

- Add one cup of berries or chopped apples to oatmeal or hot porridge with walnuts and cinnamon. For a savory porridge, add two cups of your favorite chopped leafy greens and two cups of cooked butternut squash with sautéed garlic and onion.

- Cut up some raw veggies like cucumbers, carrots, and bell peppers. Enjoy with hummus, salsa, or guacamole and your favorite crackers. If you find eating raw vegetables uncomfortable or you don't like them, you can roast some asparagus, broccoli, cauliflower, bell peppers, and potatoes to dip instead.

- Chop up fruit and keep them in glass containers in the fridge for easy grab-and-go options.

- Each day, look in your fridge and pick at least one color in *addition to green* to incorporate into your meals.

- Add a handful of fresh chopped herbs such as parsley, dill, basil, or cilantro to your prepared salad or cooked meal.

By incorporating these three strategies, you can eat a balanced diet filled with plenty of variety over a week. You don't have to apply all strategies in every single meal or into every single day. You will get different nutrients and vitamins as you go. Remember to be easy on yourself when you get busy and don't have time to cook. Or you eat a protein bar for breakfast instead of your green smoothie. This is all great! As you become more mindful about what you eat, you will naturally include lots of nutritious green and colorful foods throughout the week!

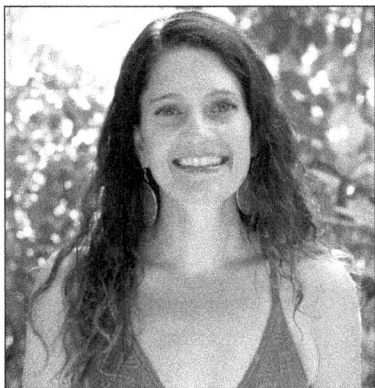

Monique Bogni, CNC, CHHC, is a certified Nutritionist and Health Coach who guides individuals in the power of food to heal and nourish their bodies. She assists her clients in transforming their diets by introducing healthier alternatives to their favorite meals. She is an expert in raw vegan cuisine and Medical Medium protocols and believes food is medicine. Monique offers a holistic and personalized approach to food, tailoring each experience to the individual's needs and encouraging them to trust their instincts to discover what truly nourishes their body, mind, and spirit.

Monique is a holistic chef who blends culinary expertise with Reiki energy healing, infusing each dish with love and intention and the finest ingredients, promoting overall well-being. She is deeply dedicated to educating others on healthy eating through her consulting, personal chef services, retreats, and cooking classes. She crafts gourmet culinary experiences and passionately creates meals that are as delicious as they are beneficial.

A Californian turned New Yorker, Monique left behind the concrete jungle with CatMan & Harley, her two indoor city cats turned jungle cats, to live on the west coast of the Nicoya peninsula of Costa Rica, one of the world's five Blue Zones. When she's not playing in the kitchen, recipe testing, or spoiling her kitties, you can find her traveling the world on a mission to eat at *all* of the healthiest restaurants, walking the beach at sunset, catching up with friends, dancing to electronic dance music, wearing glitter and drinking her mold-free coffee.

Connect with Monique:

Website: https://www.moniquebogni.com/

Facebook: https://www.facebook.com/monique.bogni/

Instagram: https://www.instagram.com/moniquebogni/

LinkedIn: https://www.linkedin.com/in/moniquebogni/

CHAPTER 4

A LIFE TRANSFORMED

FOOD AS MEDICINE FOR METABOLIC HEALTH AND DIABETES PREVENTION

Marina Vaysbaum, Rph, CHC

MY STORY

It was July of 1989, and I was 13 years old when my family and I stepped outside as refugees on American soil, leaving behind everything we knew and loved in Ukraine. It took us a long three-month journey through different countries to finally arrive at the land of opportunities. With $300 in our pocket and a few personal items, we faced the daunting prospect of starting over from scratch. I was taken away from my best friend, first love, home, the beautiful city of Odessa, my childhood, and everything that made me a happy teenager. Little did I know the stress my parents experienced during this transition, all in the name of a better future for their only child.

And so, our hardship for survival began. My father found a job washing dishes in a local restaurant while my mom worked part-time cleaning a beauty salon. Despite their challenges, my mom bravely decided to return to school to learn English and eventually enroll in a nursing program to pursue the American dream.

As for me, the transition to American life wasn't easy. I helped my mom clean the salon on weekends and cried myself to sleep most nights. It was a time of isolation, disappointment, lack of interest in life, deterioration in education and reading, and I felt like I was losing myself. This time was undoubtedly the darkest and most difficult period of my life, and I think my parent's lives as well, although I never got to ask them.

I can still vividly recall the long nights spent crammed onto a worn mattress with both of my parents. We found it abandoned on the street—a symbol of our desperate circumstances. Each night, as my mother's tears silently soaked the pillow, I felt the weight of her stress and depression pressing down on all of us. It was a heartbreaking scene that played out night after night, a constant reminder of the struggles we faced.

I'm eternally grateful to this amazing country for providing us with the opportunity and financial assistance during the first few years. I started working at 14 years old as a part-time clerk in a hospital and, after, a secretary in the real estate office, where I worked even when I started college. Despite our low-paying jobs and reliance on welfare and food stamps programs, we still struggled financially. Back in Ukraine, even though we were poor, my mom would go to the farmer's market and buy the freshest food possible, a luxury we took for granted. Little did we know that there were other kinds of food in the world, like cereal and processed foods, antibiotic-rich poultry and meat, and farmed fish. In America, the supermarket became a fun escape from our struggles and nostalgia. With limited funds, we opted out for the cheapest choices and most exciting foods—colorful cereals, crackers, potato chips, fruit juices loaded with artificial coloring, and budget-friendly meats. It was a whole new world of choices and flavors that helped distract me from homesickness. Oh, the joy of discovering new foods and experiencing the simple pleasure of grocery shopping on a tight budget!

As a few years passed, my life became a blur of busyness, stress, and suboptimal relationships. I was so consumed with work, school, and living in a bubble without looking beyond my surroundings that I forgot to stop and take a moment to breathe, appreciate the beauty of the world around me, and truly connect with the people I loved. And in this hectic, autopilot life, I lost sight of what truly mattered—living life to the fullest with joy and love in my heart.

And then, one day, my mom came to my room with tears streaming down her cheeks. "Marina, I need to tell you something," she said with a trembling voice. As I looked up from my high-school homework, I sensed the heaviness in her voice. "Lately, I have been feeling off with constant thirst, frequent urination, and general tiredness. I went to the doctor and just got a call informing me that my sugar levels are through the roof. I have diabetes and didn't even know it!" At just 42 years old, my mom's world turned upside down.

I was 16 years old and thought: *Diabetes is not that dangerous. After all, many people are living with this disease and are managing it, and besides, my mom is getting old already, so there is no need to panic.*

My teenage mind's perception was that people in their early forties are already considered old.

Another few years flew by, and I received an acceptance letter into pharmacy school. The irony is that I have no clue why I even chose that path. My life was dull and superficial, lacking passion, purpose, and ambition. School came easy to me, and I cruised through it, doing well with minimum effort. The truth was nothing truly sparked my interest. So, I settled on a profession that seemed respectable enough to please my parents.

Meanwhile, as my mom bravely fought against her relentless disease, she was bombarded with an array of medications that only seemed to add to her suffering. The disease mercilessly advanced, leaving her body ravaged and broken. I felt helpless, watching her vibrant self fade away. Each day brought a new wave of debilitating symptoms—weight gain, hair loss, high blood pressure, kidney disease, heart disease, swelling of her feet, chronic fungal infection of her skin, and probably many more conditions I don't remember.

My mom was a warrior. Despite her dream of becoming a nurse being cut short, her spirit didn't waiver. She found a job as a salesperson in a Russian bread store and traveled with my dad on cruise ships, exploring the wonders of Europe.

As her health declined and each step became more difficult, she continued to push herself. In 1998, I got married; a year later, I earned my pharmacist diploma, and in 2000, I welcomed my first daughter, Michelle. My mom took the stroller and walked with her granddaughter for hours, a testament to her unwavering love and strength. Two years later, Sonia came into our lives, and my mom's love and support only grew stronger. Though her body was failing her, her spirit remained unbroken. She may not have been able to walk as far as before, but she was always there to lend a helping hand and share in the joys of motherhood.

As time passed, my mom's legs swelled to an alarming degree, causing her skin to blister and crack. Even the slightest touch would result in open sores that wouldn't heal. At some point, she had multiple large ulcers on her feet that were painful to look at. Despite visiting numerous clinics, we found no relief. A doctor recommended doing a promising hyperbaric oxygen treatment, which wasn't covered by her insurance, but we still went for it and did a few sessions. Mom's wound started to heal.

On March 7, 2006, just a few days before her 55th birthday, she called me early in the morning, her voice trembling with fear. "Marina, I don't know what to do. I feel like I can't breathe, and each step is a struggle." My heart sank as I listened to her words. I called 911 immediately, my hands shaking as I tried to keep calm.

She was rushed to a Brooklyn hospital, where doctors ran numerous tests and scans, but despite their efforts, they couldn't find a diagnosis. I stood by her side in the ER, my heart heavy with worry. *Please, God, give doctors the wisdom to find out what's wrong and bring her back to life.* I left briefly to take my daughters to their dance class while my dad was by her side.

But then the call came. My dad's voice was strained, his words heavy with sorrow. "Please drive to the hospital as soon as possible. Mom got up to go to the bathroom and collapsed. She is unconscious." Panic gripped me as I raced back to the hospital, my mind filled with a million terrifying thoughts.

But it was too late. By the time I arrived, my mom had already slipped away, leaving me with a gaping hole in my heart that would never fully heal. It turned out she had a blood clot in her lungs, and the simple act of standing up caused it to move, leading to her tragic death. The pain of losing her so suddenly, so unexpectedly, was a weight I would carry for the rest of my days. The tears streamed down my face, and my heart shattered into a million pieces as I said my final goodbye to the woman who had been my rock, my confidante, my everything. And in that moment, the world seemed a little darker and colder without her light to guide me.

Mom's love still finds me. She sent me a miracle—a son I named in her honor. I feel that a piece of her came back to me, a reminder that love endures, even through loss.

As I continued working in the pharmacy setting, I was confronted with the harsh reality of patients suffering from many chronic diseases that seemed to only worsen with conventional treatments. I couldn't help but question why doctors only mask symptoms instead of addressing the root cause. *Why is our society plagued with illnesses like diabetes, heart disease, and cancer at such alarming rates? What can I do as a pharmacist, a wife, a mother, and a person to help my family and others?*

I refuse to accept the fate of my mother and grandmother, who left this world far too soon. So, I went on a mission to educate and empower myself and to inspire others to take control of their health and well-being. Together, we can uncover the secrets of our modern world that are making us sick and pave a path toward a brighter, healthier future.

THE SKILL

WHY WHAT YOU EAT MAKES A DIFFERENCE

In a mere blink of an eye, the rates of obesity and diabetes have soared to unprecedented levels within just one generation. Shockingly, 40% of adults and 19% of children in the United States are now classified as obese. The question that begs to be answered is: why is our generation plagued with such alarming rates of illness? How is it possible that our children are now suffering from diseases like fatty liver and diabetes, conditions that were virtually unheard of in children in the past?

Throughout human history, diabetes and obesity have been rare occurrences. Childhood obesity and type 2 diabetes were practically nonexistent. People nourished themselves with wholesome, nutrient-dense foods, and obesity was a rarity. However, as our society evolved, so too did the prevalence of obesity, diabetes, and other chronic diseases.

The development of ultra-processed foods began in the early 20th century, driven by industrialization and a need for longer-lasting convenient food. After World War II, the demand for quick, cheap meals grew as more women entered the workforce. Food companies responded by creating highly processed, packaged foods with artificial ingredients, preservatives, and flavor enhancers to improve taste and shelf life. Over time, these foods became a staple in modern diets despite their links to health issues like obesity and chronic diseases.

But the scary part is the food companies that developed ultra-processed foods stripped away our control over what we eat! Ever wonder why you can't stop at just one chip or cookie? Those foods were designed to hack your brain! Scientists carefully craft these foods with the perfect mix of sugar, fat, and salt to make them more palatable and to light up your brain like fireworks. This dopamine party makes you crave more and more. Your brain starts to think: *This stuff is amazing; give me more!* But the problem is, these foods are low in nutrients and high in empty calories, leaving you unsatisfied yet reaching for another bite.

Did you know that countries like the United Kingdom, Ireland, Sweden, Norway, Chile, and South Korea have implemented strict regulations to limit children's exposure to ultra-processed food advertisements, especially on children's TV networks? Unfortunately, many countries, including the US, still allow kids to be bombarded with junk food ads that are shown on networks like Nickelodeon and Cartoon Network. These ads make our kids vulnerable to the addictive nature of unhealthy foods.

Now, let's dive into what ultra-processed foods *really* do to our bodies and how we can take control of our health!

1. Diabetes: Eating too much sugar and refined carbs (like white bread and sugary cereals) makes our blood sugar spike. If this happens too often, our bodies stop responding to insulin, the hormone that helps control blood sugar. That's how Type 2 diabetes develops. This disease, if left unmanaged, causes heart problems, kidney damage, vision loss, and nerve damage, and makes it harder for your body to fight infections and heal any wounds.

2. Fatty Liver Disease: This disease is silently damaging millions of livers, and most people don't even know they have it. The liver is a crucial organ in removing toxins and processing nutrients from food, but when fat builds up from eating excess sugar, refined carbs, high fructose corn syrup, and processed fats, it becomes inflamed, scarred, and can develop into cirrhosis, which is irreversible and can

lead to liver failure or cancer. Fatty liver can increase the risk of Type 2 diabetes and heart disease and can make us feel tired and weak.

3. Mental Health Problems: Yes, what we eat can even affect our mood and mind! Studies show that eating ultra-processed foods can increase the risk of depression, anxiety, and mood swings. Why? These foods mess with gut bacteria that communicate with our brain and help us feel good. When they're out of balance, so are we. These damaging foods can overstimulate kid's brains, leading to hyperactivity, trouble focusing, and mood swings. For children with ADHD, ultra-processed foods can worsen symptoms, making school and daily life even harder to manage.

TAKING ACTION

There's good news: we have the power to protect ourselves and our kids from diseases linked to ultra-processed foods. By choosing whole, natural foods, we're giving our bodies the nutrients they need to stay strong and healthy. The simplest way to avoid ultra-processed foods is to focus on whole foods that don't need labels, like fresh fruits, vegetables, pasture-raised poultry, grass-fed meats, whole grains, nuts, and seeds.

One of the most impactful skills you can develop is to recognize and limit added sugars in your diet. Added sugars can hide in many surprising foods like sauces, salad dressings, and even bread. Check nutrition labels for words like "cane sugar," "high fructose corn syrup," "maltose," "dextrose," and "corn syrup." Remember that every four grams of sugar on a nutrition label equals one teaspoon of sugar. So, if a product lists 16 grams of sugar per serving, that means you're consuming four teaspoonfuls of sugar in just one portion!

Did you know that the order in which you eat your food plays a huge role in how your body processes sugar? Starting with fiber-rich vegetables, followed by protein, and ending with carbs can help slow sugar absorption. This order supports a steadier blood sugar response, avoiding the spikes that lead to energy crashes. Next time you're in your favorite restaurant, start with salad or roasted veggies, then enjoy the main course with some protein, maybe a nice piece of fish, chicken, or steak, keeping things balanced and satisfying. Finally, save the bread or pasta for last, letting carbs make a delicious appearance without causing a sugar rollercoaster. If you follow this order, you're much more likely to walk out feeling great without any post-meal energy crash!

And once you finish your delicious meal, consider going for a walk or engage in gentle movement. When you move after a meal-even something as simple as a 10-15 minute walk, it signals your muscles to absorb glucose from your blood, keeping your blood sugar levels more balanced. Think of it as helping your body clear the dinner table faster, avoiding that sluggish post-meal slump.

In contrast, moving before dinner, while it's still fantastic for general health, may not have the same benefits for blood sugar. So next time you're tempted to sink into the couch after dinner, consider a little stroll instead, which can help your metabolism and be a relaxing way to end your day! And if you add regular weight-lifting to your routine, you're really supercharging your body! Building muscle not only strengthens your body but also transforms it into a metabolism powerhouse. Muscles naturally burn more calories, even at rest, which means better blood sugar regulation even when you're just relaxing. Together, post-meal walks and strength training are the ultimate tools for boosted metabolism, steady energy, and a sense of unstoppable strength.

The shift to becoming a healthier nation is already happening. More people are understanding the harm of junk food and demanding better options, pushing big food companies to rethink their products. Every time we choose healthier foods, we're part of a movement for better health for ourselves and the next generation.

I've had the honor of working with so many inspiring people on their journey to better health, helping them manage weight, diabetes, and other chronic conditions that once seemed overwhelming. I want to share the story of Aleksei, a 45-year-old Ukrainian-born man, husband, and father. A little more than a year ago, he was at his lowest point, struggling with excess weight, fatigue, constant thirst, and irritability after years of busy construction work filled with quick meals, including soda, burgers, and pizza. For years, he ate whatever was available nearby, only having homemade meals on weekends. Then, the news hit: Aleksei was diagnosed with type 2 diabetes, and his blood glucose levels were dangerously high. His doctor told him it was a chronic, progressive disease and started him on three different medications. Heartbroken, Aleksei followed the medical plan but didn't feel any better, even after a year on medication.

When we met, I reassured him, "Don't lose hope; you can still regain control of your health. Type 2 diabetes is a nutritional disease, and it's within your power to manage and even reverse it through diet and lifestyle changes." I created a nutrition plan tailored to his needs, along with some key supplements to address deficiencies and calm inflammation. The change was astounding. Within a week, Aleksei's blood sugar began to stabilize, and within a month, he no longer needed medication. Today, he's healthier, happier, and filled with a level of energy he can't remember feeling before.

Seeing someone take charge of their health like Aleksei did is why I love what I do. It's not just about managing a disease; it's about restoring life, energy, and joy and setting an example for future generations. My journey as a health coach has deep roots; I do this in memory of my mom, whose life was taken too soon by complications from diabetes. Every person I help and every step we take towards better health is a way of honoring her and ensuring other families don't have to experience the same loss. With the right support, encouragement, and knowledge, there's always hope for a healthier future.

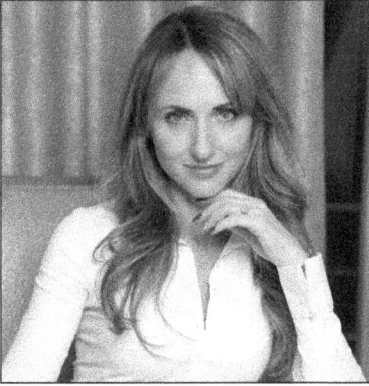

Marina Vaysbaum, Rph, CHC, is a registered pharmacist with over 20 years of experience, a dedicated health coach, and a business owner in the pharmacy industry. As a mom of three, a wife, and an unofficial home chef, she had spent years cooking wholesome meals for her family, always focused on natural ingredients. Her journey into the world of health and nutrition took a deeply personal turn when she lost her mother to diabetes at just 54, a loss that left her questioning the powerful role diet and lifestyle play in our well-being.

After facing her own health challenges, Marina immersed herself in reading and research, uncovering how deeply nutrition and stress affect our bodies. Realizing her purpose was to help others find health through sustainable lifestyle changes, she embarked on a mission to become a health coach. Through her work, she now helps individuals understand how to use food as medicine to prevent disease, find balance, and live more vibrant lives. She hopes that through knowledge and support, people can take control of their health and create a future free from preventable diseases.

Connect with Marina:

Website: https://wellnessgurucoach.com

Instagram: https://www.instagram.com/marina_wellnessguru

Facebook: https://facebook.com/marinavaysbaum

CHAPTER 5

YOU'RE GUZZLING BUT YOU'RE NOT HYDRATED

THE BEST WATER IS FOUND IN FOOD

Gina Bria, MA

MY STORY

As a young anthropologist, I never expected to stumble on a discovery that would affect so many lives and even now could support you.

THE QUESTION

I asked the simple research question: How can people living in deserts stay hydrated without eight glasses of water a day?

Everyone knows hydration depends on the volume of water intake—eight glasses a day is a baseline must, yet these communities had little to no water. How were they even alive and healthy?

It startled me to find that each desert community I studied was better hydrated than most modern people walking around with all those water bottles. *How did they do that?*

THE RESEARCH

I studied desert dwellers' total intake and discovered that the traditional foods that they ate, while different in each desert region, all had a common factor. These foods came from plants that shared a jelly-like interior, like aloe, prickly pear, and dates.

To determine what that jelly was and if it could be related to their exceptional hydration status, I tracked down the world's foremost scientist known for studying the gel-like material inside our cells. Dr. Gerald Pollack is a bioengineer at the University of Washington. When he agreed to take my call, an entirely new approach to hydration, without all that guzzling, emerged.

THE DISCOVERY

Dr. Pollack explained, "The gel-like material inside those desert plants is a form of highly concentrated water." It's a common ecological adaptation in desert regions to preserve scarce water and transform dew to gel by a simple reorganization of water molecules into tighter, more cohesive arrangements.

In fact, this concentrated water in gel form, based on findings from Dr. Pollack, is exactly the same kind of water found inside our own cells. That makes certain foods a perfect match for slipping concentrated water into our cells without transferring into the liquid state of water, and back again into gel. Transferring liquid into gel takes a lot of work by our cells and can even account for why guzzling so much water can still leave us dehydrated.

So imagine my shock to find that foods can hydrate better than liquid! To me, this finding was so important, not to mention a relief that we no longer have to guzzle all that water, that I've spent the rest of my career sharing foods that can hydrate better than liquid.

THE SKILL

I'm not saying we don't need to drink some water. I *am saying we can bring down the volume of liquid we're using* by partnering with specific foods and, in the process, become better hydrated. Our bodies use both kinds of water (liquid and gel) to hydrate, but in our culture, we're missing the power of sponge-like absorbing foods in our hydration formula. In fact, it's a better strategy for hydration and health because a high intake of liquid can flash flood our system, washing out the very electrolytes and nutrients that help us absorb, stabilize, and distribute hydration throughout all our cells and tissues.

THE IMPORTANCE OF HYDRATION

Every single system inside our bodies depends on hydration, starting with our brain matter, made of 80% gel water. Even a two percent loss of hydration affects the brain's cognitive capacity. Ever heard of brain fog? It's more accurately described as dehydration of vital brain cells. Our lungs, also 80% water, experience ease of breathing based on how hydrated they are. Our blood circulation and oxygenation are a vast fluid system requiring hydration to flow. Digestion and nutrient extraction depend on the solvent properties of water. Our waste remove through lymph and elimination systems all require adequate hydration to work well. Even our eyesight depends on hydration for precise focusing.

Therefore, the quality of our hydration determines our true health and longevity, yet we're only told to drink ever more, leaving behind the necessary, secret, sustaining magic of concentrated water locked in our foods.

Surely Mother Nature designed more than one way to hydrate. After all, animals also hydrate through their food. Believe it or not, cows, sheep, and horses out there grazing all day are claiming the hydration locked inside grass, which is 90% water. We think they're just munching out there, but that eating is mostly hydrating, bringing in nutrients and minerals with just the right proportion of water to dissolve the particles. This is hydration and nutrients, again perfectly proportioned, packaged by nature.

We must rethink how we're hydrating and include food in our calculations because this gel form of water dissolves and releases the nutrients it carries. That means efficient, bioavailable water, better absorbed by our cells, with no run-off. A perfect example is an apple. An apple is above 90% water, comes with a balance of electrolytes and nutrients, and has fiber and pectin for slow release, a natural drip-drip method of saturation, which I'm sure our cells and tissues appreciate. Now you know why you can say an apple is nature's perfect water bottle.

ONE MORE STORY

Before I share my list of foods, I want to tell one more story. It will start with a desert tribe in the remote Sierra Madres of Chihuahua, Mexico. The

Tarahumara are famed for their ability to run 50-mile marathons. This is a favorite pastime where the community gathers, and bets are placed, not for who will finish, as they all do, but for who helps everyone along the most, the most community-spirited runner. Here's the remarkable part. It's documented as far back as the 1600s that they're only fueled for these long-distance runs by about two tablespoons of chia seeds mixed with a little corn beer.

What I haven't shared yet is that there is a very personal side to this story affecting my own family. You'll recognize the very human, almost comic coincidences of what unfolded. While doing this research, much of it at Columbia University in New York City, I also cared for my aging mother, who lived in a residence home in Michigan. My brother and sister lived nearby and provided constant care so I, therefore, could continue my research. But I still got phone calls from my family that my mother had been hospitalized, yet again, for another incident of chronic dehydration.

Imagine my dismay and hurt while I'm sitting there in the library, often very late at night, holding an old falling-apart book about some distant tribe that described the very solution my mother needed. Not another saline IV, but a long-sustaining gel food for gentle hydration. *How could I help her from so far away?*

My solution was to grind up chia seeds in my coffee grinder, package it up, and send it to her residence, asking the nursing staff to stir a tablespoon into her morning orange juice. This simple trick was enough to secure her hydration, and until her death at 98, she was spared further hospitalization.

Do pass on this vital information to those you know who are caring for their elderly. Or our young athletes—can you imagine fueling all our after-school athletic programs with this strategy, minus the corn beer, of course? We all need better hydration strategies beyond that ever-present water-chugging advice. Even tipping a teaspoon of chia seed into that water bottle will dramatically shift how that water is absorbed.

FOODS THAT HYDRATE

Of course, after my research and experiences, chia is first on my list. Not only because the Tarahumara use it, and my mother responded, but because I actually had it tested and confirmed in Dr. Pollack's laboratory. It is indeed concentrated gel water. You, yourself, can do the experiment by dropping chia seeds in a glass of water. Watch the gel form before your very eyes. You'll note that I sent my mother ground-up chia seed. There's a reason for that. If you grind chia seed, as the Tarahumara also do, it's easier to mix in liquids or add to other foods. As my mother had diverticulosis, no doctor was about to let whole seeds near her. Grinding was a perfect workaround.

Let me give you my favorite chia recipe, especially gentle for kids and elders. I make a chia pudding, which is an excellent way to hydrate. This is a great hydration strategy if you're trying to avoid waking up at night to pee because you're ingesting gel, not flash-flooding liquid.

All the ingredients in this recipe work together to make it more than the sum of its ingredients. This recipe is from my book *Quench*, co-authored with Dr. Dana Cohen, MD, where we offer over 50 recipes and a 5-Day Plan to Optimal Hydration.

Hydrating Chia Pudding

One can full fat, coconut milk

5 tablespoons chia seeds, whole or ground as you prefer

2 generous pinches of good quality sea salt, about 1/8th teaspoon

You can sweeten the pudding to your own taste, if you like, with a little honey, maple syrup, jam, or chopped dates.

Simply place ingredients in a bowl, mix thoroughly, and remix again five to ten minutes later to avoid lumping. Eat when it thickens to your liking. It stores well in the refrigerator and will be all eaten long before you have to worry about expiration.

Besides chia seed, here's five more foods that are used in traditional cultures for hydration:

Hot Chocolate

This strategy is spread throughout South America, but especially in dry high-altitude environments like the Andes, where hydration becomes essential. Use organic natural cocoa, not the processed junk. For even more synergized impact, make it with coconut milk and a pinch of sea salt. Sweeten with honey or maple syrup.

Bone Broth

Bone broth is a classic recovery medicine famed for its gelatin content. It's used widely in traditional cultures during colds or illnesses to keep systems flowing, but everyday use will especially relieve aching muscles and stiff joints. I confess I gave up making it myself since hauling beef bones around in my backpack while shopping just wasn't practical. Thankfully, we now have quality powdered forms widely available.

Tip a tablespoon in your morning coffee.

Honey

Yes, this revered ingredient is a hydrating gel. It's universally used as a soothing agent for the throat and respiratory tract. Simply by adding honey to your tea, you've increased the tea's ability to hydrate your cells.

Coconut

In all its forms, milk, water, or even flakes, coconut releases gel similar to chia seed. Its widespread use in tropical environments brings hydration protection in hot climates. Thank you Mother Nature for the many ways you hydrate us.

Vegetables and Fruits

Finally, fruits and veggies are verifiable hydrators, as they have this same concentrated water inside their own cell structure, creating easier absorption than liquid water on its own. All fruits and veggies are more than 80% gel water! Raw or cooked, they'll increase your hydration, partnering with liquids in synergistic ways. Think soups, stews, and gazpachos for much better hydration than plain water. Even adding sliced cucumbers or blueberries to your water bottle will change how much water you absorb.

It's time to rethink guzzling water and hydrate like Mother Nature intended.

Happy hydration!

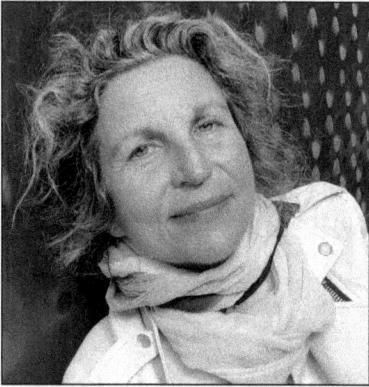

Gina Bria is an anthropologist and founder of the Hydration Foundation, recognized as a leading resource for hydration science and education. Named a Real World Scholar, she produced the first International Hydration Solution Summit and the TEDx talk: How to Grow Water: It's not Only Blue: It's Green. Bria is co-author with Dr. Dana Cohen, MD, of *QUENCH: Your Five-Day Plan to Optimal Hydration*, with 50 recipes, now in seven languages and recommended by The New York Times, Oprah's *O Magazine*, NPR, and many other media sources. Her Rehydrate Our Thirsty Mother Earth Project was selected for the Buckminster Fuller Design Science Ten-Year Award to spread better water solutions. With her colleague and filmmaker, Maxi Cohen, she's at work on a traveling Water Museum called A Movement in Water, an immersive art and science exhibit, to raise reverence and understanding of our most precious material and what all life is made from—water. She is the creator of the first-ever in-flight facial for air travel, DewGo.

Connect with Gina:

Website: www.hydrationfoundation.org

Instagram: @hydrationdaily

Hydration coaching: gina@hydrationfoundation.org

CHAPTER 6

DECODING YOUR SYMPTOMS BASED ON CROSS-REACTIVITY

HOW MOLECULAR MIMICRY CAN CAUSE MAYHEM

Stephen Cohen, DAOM, LAc

MY STORY

If you've ever observed a child hold their breath until they turn blue, almost faint, and start breathing again, it can be very traumatizing.

The sound of my son's labored breathing tore through me and reminded me of my childhood struggles. However, the wheezing of a three-year-old boy who didn't meaningfully benefit from medicine or supplements was emotionally taxing in itself. He didn't complain and didn't want to eat or do much. He was always a petite baby and started having episodes of cyanotic breath-holding. We learned how to let him work through the breath-holding, but the wheezing was a new and, as we found out, unrelated symptom.

I had my own experience with wheezing and asthma. As a child, I frequently had respiratory infections and asthmatic episodes that changed many aspects of my day-to-day life. My parents rearranged my room to help quell my allergies to dust and feathers. They installed linoleum flooring, removed toys, and frequently cleaned the room. I needed to stay inside mostly and was precluded from school recess. My second-grade teacher and

I played Neil Diamond albums in the classroom while the other children played outside.

I often gasped trying not to panic as my asthma attack started. My pediatrician in the mid-1970s convinced my mother I'd "grow out of it." Worse still, he refused to prescribe an inhaler because he thought asthma was lung weakness. He hypothesized (at my expense), "Each attack will make you stronger." When the attacks were horrible, my parents put me in the shower, hoping the hot steam would open my airway. I don't recall that ever working, and I much preferred cool air to hot. Inevitably, we rushed to the emergency room, where I was injected with adrenaline. My parents never complained about taking me to the hospital at all hours of the night, even when they had to work in the morning. Nevertheless, I felt horrible and guilty that I couldn't get more robust and live up to the pediatrician's expectations.

When I was eight, we moved into my parents' dream home. I started to play outside more and had additional experience to manage my asthma. I learned that when an attack came, I should go off by myself and quietly sip the air until the attack subsided. Little sips of air were enough to get me through the attack if I lay almost still. I identified patterns and noticed predictable triggers. For example, the first time in the summer, getting into a swimming pool—attack. Any quick transitions of temperature—attack. Racing my bicycle as hard as I could—attack. Over time, I processed the asthma and worked through it faster and faster. Looking back, I wish my pediatrician knew that there were other causes of asthma, e.g., gluten intolerance. Then, my family could've been empowered to make better food choices for me to reduce my struggles.

Except for my son's episode when he was three, I rarely thought of my asthma. Seldom would I have any signs of wheezing. I also didn't suffer from respiratory infections more than anyone else I knew. In early 2020, the world started to struggle with COVID. Despite the warnings of the virus disproportionately affecting people with preexisting health problems, I would've never included myself in that category. I was an amateur cyclist and competed in 100-mile-long races. I trained for my next long-distance race every morning in the cold, asthma-free and gluten-free.

In March 2020, just like many people, I spiked a fever. That fever turned into a cough, and that cough turned into a problem. I started to have an asthma-like attack that wouldn't end. I was blessed that I was supported by loving caregivers who cared for me and worked on treatment strategies beyond the option of hospitalization, intubation, and ventilation. I stayed home with the grace of my wife and son. I lay on my stomach for days and sipped air just like when I was a child. Sometimes, the sips were more accessible than at times when it was more challenging. Sometimes, the sips felt like an elephant was sitting on the straw I was desperate to breathe through. Perhaps going to the hospital for treatment would've been the more prudent option. We lived on the East side of Manhattan, just a few blocks from several hospitals, and I heard the news on the television of the daily death rate increasing, seemingly exponentially. I was more scared that going to the hospital meant certain death than staying home to work through it. If I could keep sipping air, the asthma-like attack would pass, like it did in the past.

As a child, there was an asthma attack that was worse than all of the others. One evening, shortly after bedtime, I woke up gasping, much worse than anything I ever experienced. My parents were at a neighbor's house, and my older sister was in her bedroom. Previously, if I felt an attack coming on, I could still call out for my parents to come to me. I might cough as a result, but I could vocalize. This time was different, and I couldn't get the words out. I remember jumping on my sleeping sister to wake her because I was out of breath. I don't recall much beyond her calling for help and then my parents with me in the emergency room. I don't doubt that I was administered another adrenaline injection. That was the closest I ever got to not breathing.

At the worst of my COVID experience, I awoke one night unable to breathe. There was simply no air. My lungs felt like they were filled with gelatin, and their weight was too much to move. The sipping was not enough anymore, and I felt like I had just enough oxygen to be conscious, but I was otherwise immobile. That was a dark moment. *Will I suffocate in my bed?* Each second felt like hours, and I had no more strength to sip. As I started to wish for the suffocation to be complete, a memory came to me. A teacher previously said, "People who meditate breathe and eat less." And so, I 'took my mantra' and surrendered.

When I woke hours later, I had returned to very shallow breathing and was able to have my wife call for more medical support. Eventually, and seemingly with bottles of medicine and supplements, prayers, and love, I was one of the lucky ones to get through a harrowing time. My childhood asthma, the pediatrician who wrongly made me suffer without an inhaler, and my parents and sister who cared for me as an asthmatic child all ultimately contributed and prepared me to get through my COVID-related respiratory distress.

Even without the experience of COVID-19, my early struggles with asthma haunted me as I listened to my baby boy wheeze. It began suddenly in the late summer of 2016. There was no other sign or symptom to explain why, out of nowhere, he was wheezing and mainly unresponsive to intervention. The first day he had any symptoms, I traveled to see my parents, and my wife would visit us in a few days. We just celebrated an event at home, and a dear friend went over the top and sent us countless sunflower arrangements. We had a sunflower bouquet on many surfaces in the foyer, living room, dining room, and bedrooms. Coincidentally, we recently started cooking with sunflower oil. We learned that cooking at higher temperatures with olive oil was not ideal, and we pivoted. In a loving accommodation, my mother stocked her house with sunflower oil and pre-cooked several meals.

Our son's wheezing worsened during the visit with my parents in South Carolina. We were frequently in touch with several medical providers, all trying to understand why the wheezing got worse when we were outside and after meals. *Undoubtedly, they must be related.* Several practitioners suggested that South Carolina was having a terrible ragweed season. One person informed us, "Sunflowers are in the same family as ragweed," which inspired what we learned. We looked up what other foods might be in the same family as ragweed and came upon the concept of Oral Allergy Syndrome and a table provided by the American Academy of Allergy, Asthma, and Immunology. It charted which foods cross-react with specific environmental allergies. Sure enough, we found out melon is cross-reactive with sunflowers and ragweed; at the time, our son ate plenty.

We immediately changed our son's diet to avoid every food on the cross-reactive list. Within a short period, his treatments were productive, and he stopped gasping. Soon after that, we discontinued all treatments, and his respiration was fine. That set us on a journey to understand what cross-reactivity was and whether there were any other ways we were inadvertently exposing him to problematic foods.

To help understand my health journey and that of many members of my family, I refocused my career many years before my son's birth. My wife encouraged me to leave the business world and begin the journey of an education in Eastern medicine that culminated in a clinical doctorate. I spent many years treating patients in my New York City office, supporting patients worldwide, and soaking up clinical pearls from luminaries and pioneers in the medical field. Through the complete dedication to learning how to dig to a deeper level of understanding and provide options and resources to patients struggling to find answers, I discovered that molecular mimicry and cross-reactivity were often the culprits baffling patients and clinicians alike. Learning how to decipher, test, and manage symptoms that should have been resolved but continued to persist was enhanced by listening to our son wheeze and gasp. His symptoms were caused by a similar reaction to seemingly different substances but were viewed as the same by his immune system. Helping others navigate these issues has been beyond a professional mission and a personal passion.

Many people struggle on the health continuum, from relatively simple but nagging symptoms to chronic disease. Moreover, the WHO suggests that non-communicable diseases will account for up to 86% of deaths by 2050: (https://bit.ly/3CCSKGv) Understanding how foods, chemicals, and pathogens might be viewed interchangeably by the immune system provides an opportunity to navigate around these triggers. Beyond minimizing symptoms, the lessening of the inflammatory response can have profound effects and help restore your health. Once a few key concepts are learned, the already established decoder rings become easy to navigate. Then, you're empowered to make choices and work with your doctors, clinicians, and family to improve your health!

THE SKILL

NAVIGATING THE IMMUNE SYSTEM: UNDERSTANDING ANTIBODIES

Our immune system is a vast defense network, with many types of cells working together to protect us from invaders. These cells are stationed at every entry point in our bodies and travel through our blood and other body fluids, like soldiers on guard. One essential part of this system is a group of cells called immunoglobulins, also known as antibodies.

Antibodies identify and respond to potentially harmful substances like bacteria, viruses, chemicals, or certain foods. When they detect something unusual, they can react differently, causing a fever, muscle aches, or allergic reactions like sneezing or asthma symptoms. Sometimes, we don't notice these immune responses; other times, they lead to more severe health issues.

There are five main types of antibodies, each known by a letter: IgA, IgD, IgE, IgG and IgM. Knowing which type of antibody is active helps us understand what's triggering a response and whether it's due to an allergy or something else, like an intolerance. This knowledge can guide us in creating a plan to manage symptoms.

ALLERGIES VS. NON-ALLERGIC REACTIONS

When someone is allergic to something, it's usually because their immune system's IgE antibodies react to a protein in that substance. Common allergy symptoms include itchy eyes, sneezing, and sometimes stomach pain. If an antihistamine helps relieve these symptoms, it often indicates that IgE is involved. Those allergies are frequently seasonal.

As published by the American Academy of Allergy, Asthma, and Immunology (AAAAI), the dominant seasonal pollens are:

Spring: Birch

Summer: Timothy and Orchard Grasses

Late Summer: Ragweed

Fall: Mugwort

For some people, allergies can be triggered by foods with proteins similar to these pollens. This is called cross-reactivity. For example, birch pollen can cross-react with stone fruits, like apples and cherries, so someone with a birch pollen allergy might experience symptoms when they eat those fruits, even outside of pollen season. And the reverse is true, too.

Some might experience seasonal allergy symptoms out of season because their IgE immune response to the stone fruit is as if they were exposed to the birch or tree pollen during the peak pollen season. (https://bit.ly/4ehxe79)

Another example is derived from my son. We fed him juicy, wonderful melon and cooked with sunflower oils while he was breathing in the pollen of sunflowers in the home during a heavy ragweed pollen season. The proteins of these substances are all cross-reactive with each other and overwhelmed his system, causing his symptoms. We couldn't help him overcome the wheezing until we could follow the map of allergic cross-reactivity for IgE proteins.

Non-allergic reactions, on the other hand, are often linked to different antibodies, such as IgA, IgM, or IgG. Generally, IgA is the antibody found in the body's fluids. For example, our tears, digestive, and reproductive fluids should all have IgA antibodies. Further, our body circulates IgM and IgG to enhance our defense system with IgA. The IgM is more of an immediate response to fight an active infection or protein associated with such a disease. The IgG is more of a long-term antibody that remains vigilant to seemingly foreign proteins.

These antibodies may respond to foods, chemicals, or infections, but instead of causing classic allergy symptoms, they can lead to sensitivities or intolerances. For example, eating certain foods, like those containing gluten or dairy, might cause digestive discomfort without sneezing or itching as in traditional allergies. Understanding which antibody is causing the reaction is critical to identifying what's causing the problem.

CROSS-REACTIVITY AND MOLECULAR MIMICRY

Cross-Reactivity

As in the case of birch and stone fruits, as well as pollen and melon, cross-reactivity occurs when the immune system recognizes similar proteins in different substances and reacts to both as if they were the same.

Molecular Mimicry

Molecular mimicry is similar, but it is when the immune cells can't distinguish between the foreign protein and our own body. In molecular mimicry, an antibody created in response to an external substance (like a bacteria, virus, or specific food proteins) may also confusingly target similar proteins in the body's tissues, triggering an autoimmune reaction.

For example, antibodies that react to thyroid protein can also respond to foods containing latex hevein (e.g., banana, avocado, and kiwi).[1,2] Some proteins in these foods resemble thyroid proteins, so people with autoimmune thyroid conditions might react to these foods due to molecular mimicry. Suppose you're struggling with antibodies to your thyroid protein. In that case, you might benefit from investigating if you are also producing antibodies to cross-reactive foods or even an infection, causing molecular mimicry.

TAKING CONTROL OF YOUR HEALTH

Navigating cross-reactivity and molecular mimicry might understandably seem daunting at first. There is hope!

Like those for oral allergy syndrome, allergy cross-reactivity charts map out common cross-reactive foods and are readily available (for example, https://bit.ly/4ehxe79). They are long-established and reliable.

Investigating intolerance and sensitivities is more complicated but also very achievable. There are many resources to rely on to decode which foods, chemicals, or infections might be cross-reacting to the human tissue, causing or contributing to your symptoms. Armed with the knowledge of why you feel the way you do, you become empowered to move forward to resolve your symptoms and become well again.

---

1 Kharrazian, D., Herbert, M., & Vojdani, A. (2017). Immunological Reactivity Using Monoclonal and Polyclonal Antibodies of Autoimmune Thyroid Target Sites with Dietary Proteins. Journal of thyroid research, 2017, 4354723. https://doi.org/10.1155/2017/4354723

2 Radauer, C., Adhami, F., Fürtler, I., Wagner, S., Allwardt, D., Scala, E., Ebner, C., Hafner, C., Hemmer, W., Mari, A., & Breiteneder, H. (2011). Latex-allergic patients sensitized to the major allergen hevein and hevein-like domains of class I chitinases show no increased frequency of latex-associated plant food allergy. Molecular immunology, 48(4), 600–609. https://doi.org/10.1016/j.molimm.2010.10.019

NEXT ACTION STEPS:

Allergies:

1. Recognize that there may be more than one cause.

2. Use a cross-reactivity reference guide.

3. Once you know the additional offenders, try avoiding these foods and see if that improves your symptoms.

4. Consider additional allergy testing and treatment for the suspicious allergens.

Autoimmune and Other Conditions Associated with Abnormal Levels of Antibodies:

1. Understand that an underlying trigger often causes the immune system to escalate and inadvertently attack our tissues.

2. Using the known elevated antibody as a starting point, use a reference guide or a professional consultation to understand cross-reactive foods, chemicals, and pathogens (viruses, bacteria, fungus, etc).

3. Create a plan to manage these triggering exposures and associated reactions.

4. Similarly to allergies, you can work with your clinician to look into testing for any molecular mimicry that might allow for a more detailed diagnosis and treatment plan.

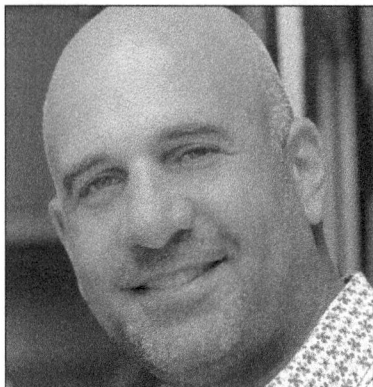

Stephen Cohen, DAOM, LAc, is the founder of AXIOM Holistic and a nationally board-certified and state-licensed acupuncturist with extensive training in both Eastern and Western medical traditions. After a successful career in the corporate world, Stephen transitioned to East Asian medicine following his own transformative experience with acupuncture and herbology.

Stephen's approach is rooted in uncovering the true causes of illness rather than simply treating symptoms. As a tireless advocate for his clients, he supports and challenges the status quo while collaborating with other healthcare teams. He integrates his expertise in Traditional Chinese Medicine, Japanese acupuncture techniques, Trigger Point Dry Needling, and other healing modalities to help patients achieve lasting health and balance.

Stephen has advanced training in autoimmune disease, fertility and reproductive health, sports medicine, vocal health, and internal conditions. His holistic and integrative approach tailors treatment to each individual's needs, drawing from years of clinical experience and rigorous education. This includes advanced studies in Oncology Acupuncture at Memorial Sloan-Kettering Cancer Center and Acupuncture for Labor and Delivery at Lutheran Hospital.

In addition to his clinical work, Stephen consults with pharmaceutical companies to explore drug formulation and application, bridging Eastern and Western approaches to health. He is also a guest speaker on a range of health topics.

Stephen is licensed in New York and South Carolina and is committed to helping patients heal and live with greater vitality and balance. He resides in Florida with his family and enjoys tennis and cycling in his free time.

Connect with Stephen:

Website: https://www.axiomholistic.com

CHAPTER 7

GOOD AND FREE

OVERCOMING FOOD OVERWHELM WITHOUT FOMO

Amy Levine Cohen, MA
mindbodygreen Functional Nutrition Expert

MY STORY

"I never want you to experience what it feels like as a kid to feel sick and be told it's in your head," I said to our son growing in my womb. "I will instill a sense of trust for you to know your body," I vowed. "From a very young age, you will instinctively know when something is truly off." I didn't want what happened to me to be something he would ever experience.

It was a hot summer day. I'm 12 and at sleepaway camp for the fifth year in a row. Curled up in a ball on the bottom bunk, agonizing pains ripped through my stomach while everyone else was free, having fun, playing sports, dancing, and doing arts and crafts. Days, and then weeks (for hours on end), I suffered. I called my parents from the camp office, "Please come get me and bring me home," I begged. My dad did his best to understand what was going on. My mom thought I was concocting a story. "It was your choice to be at camp; you need to stick it out until it's over."

How am I going to make it through? I have another month to go. I'll find a way to show I'm not faking it.

I elected to go with all the sick kids to the local doctor and get checked. "Mom, the doctor believes something is happening. He wants you to make an appointment with a gastroenterologist. You need to come get me." They did, and I was indeed sick with a debilitating food intolerance to lactose. I altered my diet and felt good again. Over the years, with various strategies, I overcame it.

More than two decades later, living with my boyfriend (now husband), another food intolerance crept into our lives. For me it started with bloating and gas. For him, it was skin irritation. We knew gluten was the culprit and decided as a couple that in order for it to truly work for our bodies, it would be all or nothing based on research and medical guidance. We took the leap to go 100% gluten-free and never turned back.

Given that we both have gluten intolerance and are genetically predisposed, we decided to raise our son gluten-free as we navigated his health issues through the years. When he was two and started preschool, we sent his lunch and all his snacks to keep him safe. He knew from the get-go that he had his own special homemade or purchased treats we lovingly packed with an uplifting note. He never asked or considered that he was different because it was our norm to make sure as a family we always had delicious and fun food options as substitutes for what everyone else was getting—whether at school, a birthday party, or somewhere else. Bottom line: We created a strong support system to maintain a gluten-free lifestyle. We were in it together.

The truth is that 'safe' is only as far as can be seen. You don't know what you don't know. On one particular day, when our son was almost four, we picked him up from preschool on our way to a pre-kindergarten interview. Insisting we take gluten-free pretzels and cookies from our personal snack stash kept at school, he placed a handful of each into a white paper cup and said, "Take it Mama, for your bag."

It seemed strange at the time, however we always did trust he knew something unknown to others. With huge smiles on our faces, excited about the prospect of attending a pre-kindergarten through 12th-grade school, we checked in at the admissions table and proudly stuck our name tags to our shirts. Marching down the hall as a family of three holding hands, we got to the door where each child was whisked away to be evaluated by the teachers. *He's safe*, we thought. The parents, about 40 of us, went upstairs for a group meeting with the head of admissions. About an hour into the information session, the director informed us, "Don't worry, your kids are downstairs enjoying huge chocolate chip deli cookies."

My husband and I looked at each other in shock. Our smiles turned to jaw-dropping expressions. *OMG, they never mentioned serving food or asking us about food allergies or intolerances.* And then we remembered the white cup of gluten-free snacks taken from the preschool. We both frantically stood up as the admissions assistant elegantly sauntered into the room. I grabbed the cup from my bag and handed it off to my husband, who caught the eye of the admissions assistant. He passed it off to her, saying, "Our son has food intolerances; he can only eat these." "I'm on it," she said with urgency as she darted down the stairs.

Thankfully, an anaphylactic response wasn't a concern. We sat amongst the other parents, praying the session would soon end, knowing we couldn't be in two places at once. We wanted to stand out in a good way and be one of the few accepted to the school, not be considered high maintenance and rejected.

We've been so vigilant. How could they not have asked about food allergies? How did we not think to make mention?

The meeting ended and we rushed downstairs to the calm classroom where our son played with two other kids and two teachers. They handed us half of the huge cookie to show us how much he didn't eat. The teacher said, "He asked if it was good and free," and I told him it was. "Oh no," we said, looking at each other in disbelief. "He asked if it was gluten-free," we said simultaneously. He didn't enunciate clearly, even though he did his best to articulate his words. It was the only time he had gluten, and a mistake like that never happened again.

Through these experiences, I became a passionate advocate for gluten-free awareness, and addressing how clear communication and trustworthy support is vital. To do this, I shifted my health coaching business to work with individuals and families navigating food allergies and intolerances. I help them make the switch from gluten-full to gluten-free by eliminating overwhelm with simple solutions, showing them that fear of missing out (FOMO) doesn't need to exist and creating accountability as they learn to eat in a new way.

According to a report by Research and Markets, "The global market for food allergy and intolerance products is estimated at $36.1 billion in 2023 and is projected to reach $53.9 billion by 2030." Whether it's gluten, dairy, soy, nuts, or something else, there's a growing health need to cater to those who need to eliminate certain foods or ingredients. If you or someone you know has food allergies or intolerances, it can feel isolating. However, now that it's more of an epidemic, overwhelm doesn't need to exist when modeling values and messages, understanding how to decode labels, finding fun substitutes, asking the best questions when eating out of the house, and engaging other people in your lives to increase confidence and empowerment, supporting food choices at any age.

THE SKILL

A STRONG FOUNDATION

Structure is important when it comes to raising and working with kids. It's part of the foundation for them to have a sense of security, consistency, stability and safety. Values are also important. A value is a personal truth you want to instill in your children that is the basis for their life decisions. If you think back to your childhood, you may not remember choosing your values; they likely seemed to be part of the fabric of your life. That said, this is your opportunity to consciously share your family values and messages (including the facts) your child needs to know about allergies or intolerances they may have.

What we believe, know, and convey, how we say it, and how we show it—both verbally and nonverbally—all send strong messages to the young people in our lives as they grow up. When values and messages about health and well-being are shared and discussed in a healthy, positive, and proactive way, it helps kids to feel and become empowered. This is important for many reasons, including the goal of having them successfully take care of themselves as they navigate the world around them.

If you feel you need to do a better job sharing values and messages, know you're not alone. It's not too late to start or build a stronger foundation more intentionally. Consider what's important to your family and your child's health related to the topic you want to address—in this case, not eating a certain ingredient or food. To do this, you can take advantage or create teachable moments—opportunities to get your messages across in a loving, positive way.

Start simple and continue this process regularly:

SHARE at least one of your family values or messages of importance.

IDENTIFY and ask a question you have or illustrate a point with one or two healthy options or scenarios.

PROVIDE an opportunity for your child to share their thoughts and feelings. You can also use this as an opportunity to choose options or scenarios.

REINFORCE their situation, point of view, or decision with a positive response.

Using Gluten as an Example:

1. **Share:** It's important to take care of your body. We know gluten makes your body ache; let's only eat what makes you feel well.

2. **Identify:** When you're at the party, while kids are eating the birthday cake, you can have gluten-free cookies or gluten-free cake to enjoy.

3. **Provide:** Do you prefer gluten-free cookies or gluten-free cake?

4. **Reinforce:** That's a great choice. I'll bring that to the party.

Using Dairy as an Example:

1. **Share:** It's really important that you have snacks at school that are dairy-free.

2. **Identify:** When snacks are handed out at school, what do they give you to eat?

3. **Provide:** How do you feel that you need to eat dairy-free at school? After feelings are shared and discussed, let your child know you can both talk with the teacher about having dairy-free snacks available when the class gets their snacks.

4. **Reinforce:** Thank you for letting me know how you feel. I'm here to support you to keep your body healthy and for you to get what you need in a fun way. Then, let your child know that speaking up and having a solution is one way they can advocate for themselves.

Having these conversations as part of your usual casual conversation (and often), is one of the best ways to teach your children how to navigate their feelings, be aware of what they need, feel empowered to speak up, and say or do what they need to stay healthy.

DECODING LABELS

When needing to avoid a certain ingredient or food due to an allergy or intolerance, it's important to understand how to decode labels and share this information with your child so they learn how to do it for themselves.

- Know how the ingredient(s) you want to eliminate is listed on a product label.

- Look for the obvious words associated with what you need to eliminate.

- Learn where the ingredient you want to eliminate is commonly hidden and see if that's an ingredient.

- Find out FDA standards for what you want to avoid and see if there are certification marks on packaging that can help you spot what's safe to consume.

- Identify a trusted non-profit advocacy group that has fact sheets, blogs, etc., so you don't have to reinvent the list.

- Create a cheat sheet for you and your child to use as you look at labels together.

Let's take a closer look at gluten as an example. Gluten is a group of proteins that's in certain grains. Gliadin and glutenin are two of the common proteins. It's often used to bind ingredients together so they keep a certain shape or provide elasticity or stretchiness. Wheat, barley, rye, spelt, triticale, farro, malt, brewer's yeast, and more all contain gluten. So, when looking at a label you want to see if any of these are listed so you know to avoid that product.

Oats inherently don't contain gluten. However, there can be cross-contamination during processing. Some people who are gluten-free eat gluten-free (gf) oats. Others avoid them completely, as even gf oats contain a protein similar to gluten called avenin. This protein can trigger a similar immune response in some people, as if it were gluten.

Gluten can also be hidden in "natural flavors" on an ingredient list. Other times, ingredients like maltodextrin (commonly found on labels) can be made of wheat unless it specifically says it's derived from corn, potato, or rice.

When it comes to gluten, the U.S. Food & Drug Administration (FDA), in addition to limiting the unavoidable presence of gluten to less than 20 parts per million (ppm), allows manufacturers to label a food "gluten-free" if the food does not contain any of the following:

- an ingredient that is any type of wheat, rye, barley, or crossbreeds of these grains,
- an ingredient derived from these grains and that hasn't been processed to remove gluten or
- an ingredient derived from these grains that has been processed to remove gluten if it results in the food containing 20 or more ppm gluten.

Find more information here: https://www.fda.gov/consumers/consumer-updates/gluten-free-means-what-it-says

That said, there are third-party certifications to help consumers safely navigate gluten-free products. One of these is the distinctive mark of the Gluten-Free Certification Organization (GFCO) (learn more at https://gfco.org). The GFCO mark represents a rigorous certification process that includes verifying the product is at or below 10ppm of gluten (https://gfco.org/certification/)

When you see "gluten-free" printed on a product and/or a certification mark (know the ppm limits of the mark you like the most and what is best for your reaction to gluten), if there is a statement about being manufactured on shared equipment or in a facility that has the allergen present it needs to comply with FDA and certification mark ppm standards. Typically, companies do this as a way to cover their butt for liability in the event something goes awry in production. If you see this statement on a product that does not say "gluten-free," it's best to avoid the product.

SUBSTITUTIONS ARE ENCOURAGED

We all have our favorite foods and routines of what we prefer for our meals and snacks. Food allergies or intolerances can create overwhelm as many have the fear that they will no longer be able to have foods they love. However, many substitutions are incredibly satisfying, thanks to the new companies and products that are catering to those who need to eliminate a certain ingredient or food.

Do This Now:

To make the process easy, make a list of common foods that are enjoyed for meals, snacks, and desserts. Gluten-free or dairy-free? Check out my list of delicious substitutions that even the biggest foodies love at https://givingupglutenforgood.com, and FOMO will no longer be an issue. You can also use Google and social media to find alternatives.

EATING OUT OF THE HOUSE

It's possible to successfully eat out of the house. These days, with so many people aware of and needing to avoid certain foods, many food establishments have the details on the menu or can easily make accommodations to the order. There are a few basic questions you can research ahead of time and ask before you order to make it easier to eat out, feel safe and enjoy your meal. Teaching your child to understand and use these tips is invaluable.

- Does the food establishment have a menu with a key for your needs (gluten-free, dairy-free, vegan, vegetarian, soy-free, nut-free, seed oil-free, etc.) that makes navigating what you need easy?

- Do they have a system in place to identify dietary needs like certain shaped plates, signs for a food order that make it recognizable that it's safe (like a flag on a toothpick), etc.?

- How do they prevent cross-contamination to meet your needs? Do they have a dedicated space, equipment, and utensils, etc. to prevent cross-contamination? Ask specific questions like, do they use a dedicated fryer, for what you need?

- Did you double check with the manager or server when the food is served to be certain the order is prepared correctly related to your request?
- What else is important for you to know to feel safe?

There are also many apps available to help find appropriate restaurants. If you're gluten-free, there's Find Me Gluten Free and more. You can also google programs that provide listings. For example, Chef to Plate (CTP) is a gluten-free awareness and education effort committed to ensuring that dining out is stress-free for those living gluten-free (check out https://gluten.org/ctp). Restaurants that meet certain criteria are able to be part of the CTP directory.

TEAMWORK

In my experience, when the immediate family (at the least) supports each other as a team, rather than it only being for the person who needs to eat differently, it solidifies a strong foundation. This includes avoiding the same ingredients (when possible), coming up with solutions to challenges together, and discussing how to handle peer pressure in social situations related to allergies or intolerances. Additionally, teaching other people involved in the child's life—babysitters, nannies, grandparents, teachers, and others who have an integral role—the tips you learned from this chapter. Ultimately, you're creating an environment that supports and cares about your child's physical and emotional well-being, helping them grow up strong, healthy, confident, empowered, and able to advocate for what they need. The subsequent perk: A lifestyle that can elevate the health and well-being of all involved.

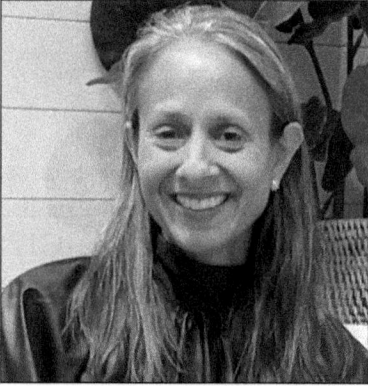

Amy Levine Cohen, MA, is a gluten-free foodie and mindbodygreen Functional Nutrition Expert. She's also a passionate gluten-free advocate, laying the groundwork with the Gluten Intolerance Group (GIG) to relaunch the Chef to Plate (CTP) program—that connects diners with restaurants serving gluten-free options (check out https://gluten.org). Her gluten-free journey started more than 15 years ago when she decided to give up gluten before it was popular. And when she did, she went all in. Amy knew in order for it to truly work for the body it had to be 100%. She took the leap and never turned back. Her family and pup are 100% gluten-free too! Over the years, Amy has truly leveled up how to eat gluten-free (and dairy-free) and enjoy every bite! She helps individuals and families realize that overwhelm doesn't have to be an ingredient when you're gluten-free. Her 5 Step Giving Up Gluten For Good Process makes it simple and can be used for other allergies, intolerances, or food preferences. Follow Amy as she shares her secrets to success and tips to love living a 100% GF DF lifestyle.

Connect with Amy:

Website: https://givingupglutenforgood.com

Instagram: https://www.instagram.com/givingupglutenforgood

CHAPTER 8

UNDERSTANDING THE BASIS OF LOVE

HOW TO FEED WITH NUTRITION AND NOT CALORIES

Sandra Cammarata, MD

MY STORY

I have been a healer for over 40 years, and I was not a good one for over half of those years. Six years of medical school, five years of adult and child psychiatric training, researching the latest papers, caring, and being empathic was not enough to make me the excellent healer I needed to be for the patients who trusted me, for my children, and for all the people I have loved and love.

My way of treating and caring was not whole; I provided only parts of a treatment. I paid attention to the symptoms I was trained to treat but missed listening to the entire story. People come to their doctors when they are suffering. They describe their symptoms, and we treat those symptoms. Then, they return to the environment that caused the symptoms with one or more pills we gave them.

Most of my patients had to take their medications for many years; it was challenging to taper them off and even harder to offer a substitute. It is not easy to convince someone who is depressed to exercise or cook a homemade meal. As a child and adolescent psychiatrist, I am well-trained in diagnosing and providing my patients with the proper medication. Still, I failed to empower my patients to participate actively in their healing.

According to the latest national survey, only twenty-seven percent of the 105 medical schools surveyed met the minimum 25 required hours of nutrition training set by the National Academy of Science. Hence, my knowledge of nutrition came from my childhood experience. I grew up in Sicily in the sixties and seventies, a world that knew no fast food. The food was whole, seasonal, fresh, and cooked from scratch. My parents worked, but dinner and lunch were served at the dinner table, and we waited for those who were not around. Meals were an offering, a daily ceremony, and a way of life.

Mark was one of many patients brought to my office by his parents because he was hyperactive, anxious, depressed, and emotionally dysregulated. He often carried a tall soda, fast food, and colorful snacks between his orange-greased fingers. He ate in the waiting room with earbuds and a screen before his hyper-focused eyes. It became clear that Mark was only one of many patients whose brains were overfed and nutritionally deficient. I was forced to pay attention to the role his diet played in the chronicity of his symptoms.

My patients' brains were inflamed not just because of genetics or environmental factors but because they lacked essential nutrients. Appropriate brain development requires, among others, adequate amounts of protein, zinc, choline, iron, folate, iodine, omega-3 fatty acids, and vitamins A, D, B6, and B12. Failure to provide these essential nutrients can result in long-term learning, behavioral, and emotional problems.

Our children are our seeds. We need to place them in good soil. The thicker the soil, the stronger the roots. We need to expose them to sunlight many hours per day, we need to keep them hydrated with clean water, we need to protect them from pesticides and other toxins, and we need to give them organic whole foods. Properly cared for, they will grow to survive hurricanes and earthquakes and anything else life throws their way, and they will grow to be fertile and bear fruits and will provide others with strength and sustenance. Unfortunately, we are not doing a good job.

Mark is not alone. Two-thirds of our children's diet comprises processed and ultra processed food, which provides excessive fats, carbohydrates, poor-quality proteins, and very few micronutrients, such as vitamins and minerals. Processed food is nutritionally deficient, obesogenic, and addictive. In 1980, seven percent of our children were obese; in 2010, eighteen percent (one in five); currently, one in three children is obese. Twenty percent of our children have been diagnosed with mental illnesses. Obesity in children is increasing exponentially, together with diagnoses of depression, ADHD, autism, anxiety, and suicide.

Fast food made it hard for Mark's brain to function well. The connection between his two brains (gut and brain) was faulty.

Yes, we have two brains, one in our skull and one in our gut.

Mark did not want to live any longer, and he gave up. A lot of his childhood was defined by poor grades, being reprimanded for poor behavior, and his inability to manage his emotions. He tried multiple medications that helped for a brief time and that had side effects he hated.

Like most American families, they ordered out often. Mark ate his food alone in his room. He abandoned sports. He did not believe he was good enough because he was made fun of by other children for being overweight, so he became more overweight. His friends were those he made playing video games online and all night. He saw no sunlight and he avoided the pool or the beach in the summer because he did not like how he looked.

Mark was disillusioned and did not want to take medications anymore. I decided to turn his giving up into a need to regain control over his life, so we made a pact. "Mark, if you can let go of fast food, we can stop some of your medications. And if you can eat six servings of fruits and vegetables a day, you can skip therapy." I told him that if he could exercise and move his body out in the sun for 20 minutes daily, he could earn 20 minutes extra in gaming. If he slept eight to nine hours every night, he could start looking at a used car for when he got his permit.

THE IMPACT OF A FAST-FOOD DIET ON OUR TWO BRAINS

Fast food contains lots of sugar, unhealthy fats, and excessive sodium and has been deprived of fiber by design. The healthy microbiome dies without adequate fiber, and we are left with less gut microbial variety, which makes our health suffer. Excessive sugar produces toxic byproducts that weaken the tight junctions among the cells lining the gut, leading to a "leaky gut." When the gut lining barrier leaks, the toxins get reabsorbed into the bloodstream, causing inflammation and other health issues. The microbiome comprises our gut's trillion bacteria, fungi, and viruses. It is our pharmacy. It makes hormones, peptides, and neurotransmitters and is integral to many other functions necessary for our metabolism and immune response. Studies show a lack of specific bacteria in the microbiomes of children diagnosed with Autism Spectrum Disorder and possibly ADHD.

New and exciting research explores which microbiome bacteria are essential for optimal mental health. A new generation of psychobiotics (friendly bacteria that reduce inflammation, manage blood sugar, reduce depression, and improve sleep) is being discovered. Hopefully, we will be able to treat some, if not most, psychiatric disorders with probiotics soon.

These friendly bacteria help produce neurotransmitters and short-chain fatty acids essential for brain health. The gut microbiome produces seventy percent of serotonin and thirty percent of dopamine, which are utilized in our body. Serotonin gives us a sense of well-being, while dopamine fuels motivation and drive. Inflammation results in an imbalance between the brain's calming GABA receptors and the excitatory glutamate receptors, leaving the brain in an excited state. A mother's nutrition during pregnancy and the first three years of her child's life is crucial for developing a healthy microbiome. Interestingly, a child's taste buds begin to be stimulated in the womb; the foods a mother prefers to eat during pregnancy can influence her child's food preference later.

MICRONUTRIENTS MATTER FOR MOOD AND BEHAVIOR

A study conducted in juvenile detention centers showed that feeding children a whole food diet decreased aggression by ninety-five percent, restrains use decreased by seventy-five percent, and suicide improved by one hundred percent. Suicide is the third cause of death in teenage boys. Supplementing juveniles with five vitamin Bs reduced aggression by twenty-eight percent. In another study, Arizona school children receiving a multivitamin supplement had forty-seven percent fewer suspensions.

A healthy diet feeds our two brains, changes behavior, improves well-being, and provides our cells with all the micronutrients necessary for optimal function. Fats and sugars need specific vitamins to be best utilized. The deficiency of vitamins makes it difficult for neurons to communicate effectively, which impairs brain function and causes behavior changes. In one study, ninety-six percent of children diagnosed with ADHD had low magnesium. Magnesium is critical for brain function and is a co-factor for several chemical reactions in the body. Vitamin B6 provides support to magnesium. Eating whole food can provide B6 and magnesium in one bite.

A poor diet is often low in iron and contributes to poor attention, lack of focus, and restless legs syndrome. Iron and ferritin deficiencies decrease blood flow to the brain, making our children feel more tired. Children with ADHD tend to have low levels of ferritin compared to children who don't.

A diet without fruits, vegetables, and proteins is low in B2, B6, B12, and folate, all essential vitamins for mental health, adrenal gland, and thyroid health. Low vitamin D has been observed in several psychiatric disorders and autoimmune diseases. Our kids don't spend enough time in the sun. When they do, they wear sunscreen that blocks the absorption of vitamin D. Only twenty-one percent of infants and twenty-six percent of toddlers have adequate amounts of vitamin D. Lack of vitamins A and C and minerals like magnesium and calcium contribute to the early onset of osteoporosis, a disease that starts in childhood.

Mark ate fast food more than three times a week, which, according to research, is correlated with the development of asthma, eczema, and rhinitis and is associated with lower math and reading scores than kids who do not. Mark did not eat fruit and vegetables because processed snacks were less readily available in his house. His brother did not like fish, so no one in the house ate fish.

OMEGA-3 FATS AND BRAIN HEALTH:

Like most American families, Mark's family ate fish less than once a month. We need fish or other Omega-3 sources at least twice weekly to get the necessary omega-3 for brain and overall metabolic health. If you or your family are vegetarian or vegan and are concerned about mercury levels, algae, nuts, and seeds, or omega-3 supplementation can be a great option. Eating fish can make your child smarter.

But be smart when choosing your fish: The acronym SMASH, sardine, mackerel, anchovies, salmon, and herring can help you choose small, oily fish high in omega 3 and low in mercury. A 2015 study showed that pregnant mothers and children who ate an adequate number of fish were protected from the adverse effects of mercury and had higher IQs, up to a nine-point increase. Children who had difficulty with reading were able to improve their reading skills after six months of supplementation with omega-3 fatty acids. Omega-3 supplementation reduces asthma symptoms, frequency of episodes, and eczema.

Supporting the Mitochondria with Omega-3s: Omega-3 fatty acids help to reduce inflammation in the body. They are necessary for maintaining a healthy mitochondria membrane. Mitochondria are our cells' organelles that produce energy (ATP). Mitochondria's health declines with age and inflammation. The brain contains the most significant amount of mitochondria compared to the rest of our body. This is not a surprise because our brain is only 2% of our body weight but uses 20% of our total energy. New research has shown that a particular group of children diagnosed with autism have specific mitochondrial defects.

Mark held his part in the deal. He left his room to go outside, and he became curious again. He tried hockey and liked it. He played increasingly and got good enough to try out for his school team. He was smiling more. He decreased his fast-food intake and reached out for fruits and vegetables when he wanted a snack. Children who eat five to six servings of fruit and vegetables are happier than those who don't. He lost fat and built muscle. He successfully came off most of his medications. He shut his phone off when he went to sleep, and because of it, his cortisol level went down at night, and he slept better. His focus and motivation improved, and he made one good friend. He decided that life was worth living, after all.

THE SKILL

TAKING ACTION: NUTRITIONAL STEPS FOR PARENTS

Very often, when asked to make a change, it feels scary. We see changes as entering unknown territory where bad things can happen. We set big goals, and when we cannot accomplish them all, we experience failures. We are scared that we will not be able to survive without what we were asked to let go of. We fear we will not succeed; like Mark, we want to give up.

Often, the problem is not information but execution. Setting small and attainable goals is an excellent way to start making changes we can sustain.

As we discovered in this chapter, we need every vitamin, mineral, fat, carbohydrate, and protein that nature has so generously provided for us for all the cells in our body to function well, for our gut to produce what we need, and for our brain to feel awake, motivated, and happy. So, become your child's role model and change your eating habits. Children pay more attention to what you do than what you say.

Here are a few steps to get started:

1. Opt for Whole, Minimally Processed Foods with Little Added Sugar and Read Labels: Foods marketed for children have excessive amounts of sugar. Many breakfast cereals have more sugar than sodas. Read labels. Even added sugar is often found in yogurt, granola bars, and fruit juice.

2. Incorporate Good, Essential Fats: Dietary fats help kids absorb vitamins and make them feel satiated longer. Good fats are necessary for hormone production. We have learned that Omega-3s are good fats. If your child or your family does not eat fish, you can add a tablespoon of fish oil to a fruit smoothie daily. Carlson is a reliable company that makes liquid fish oil without mercury and flavors it for children.

Alpha-linoleic acid (ALA) is another critical omega-3 fatty acid in seeds and nuts. Mixed nuts are excellent snacks. Add pumpkin, flax, and chia seeds to a smoothie.

Make extra virgin olive oil your preferred cooking and dressing fat. Despite some controversy about olive oil and smoking points, a study published in Acta Scientific Nutritional Health 2018 found that cooking with extra virgin olive oil at high heat is safe and more chemically stable than other commonly used oils.

If your child is not allergic to eggs, you can encourage them to eat the whole egg. It's an excellent source of choline and helpful for brain health. If your child does not have dairy allergies, choose a full-fat dairy as a good source of fat. Coconut is a good source of healthy saturated fats. Buy one at the farmers market or supermarket and have fun smashing it together!

3. Introduce Fruits and Vegetables: Not all children will love fruits and vegetables immediately. You might have to present the same vegetable ten or more times before your child accepts the new flavor and texture. Prepare it differently, adding it to soups and mash it into a smoothie.

Involve your child in fruit and vegetable preparation, and they will be more willing to try.

Make fruits accessible by keeping them over the kitchen counter or table, make vegetables easily accessible in the refrigerator, and place them in front of the less nutritious food. Make processed food unavailable.

4. A Diverse Whole-Food Diet: This ensures children get adequate micro and macronutrients and promotes a rich and diverse microbiome. Fruits and vegetables eaten in season, as do frozen fruits and vegetables, contain the most nutrition.

5. Hydration: Water should be our preferred beverage. Thirty percent of the fructose in our children's diets comes from sweetened drinks. Eliminating sodas can improve overall health and life expectancy. The phosphoric acid present in soft drinks binds magnesium and makes it less available.

6. Exercise and light exposure: Spend ten minutes outside in the sunlight before 11 a.m. to let the sun promote the natural production of melatonin. Spending time in the sun stimulates the production of vitamin D. Spending ten minutes watching the sunset light can improve sleep quality. The orange, red, and yellow light spectrum can help regulate the circadian rhythm.

Walk the farmer's market with your child, let them touch, and pick up fruits and vegetables and cook at least one meal together.

Please encourage your child to move their body for 20 minutes daily. Exercise "snacks" (one to five minutes throughout the day) can be as helpful as exercising for a one-time stretch.

7. Mindfulness: Help your child find a way to cope with distress that does not involve phone scrolling or TV watching. Examples include listening to music, walking in nature, working on a puzzle, breathing, and meditation.

8. Supplementation: Check for nutritional deficiency with the help of a trained medical provider. Your child might have a nutritional deficiency, even with a good diet, due to malabsorption, antibiotics, or poor food quality. Nutritional deficiencies are often not found in routine blood work. They can be improved through a whole-food diet or good-quality supplements.

Most importantly, try to spend time with your child by sharing a wholesome meal, taking a walk, playing and laughing, singing and dancing, and always being kind to yourself and others.

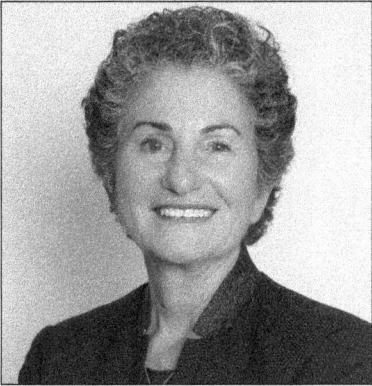

Sandra Cammarata, MD, graduated Summa Cum Laude from Catania Medical School, Italy, and specialized in General Psychiatry and Child and Adolescent Psychiatry at Tufts University in Boston. Selected in 2020 as one of Castle Connolly's "Exceptional Women in Medicine," Sandra has been practicing psychiatry in private practice in New Jersey and, since COVID, has been available for telemedicine in New Jersey and Florida. She has been awarded the Castle Connolly Best New Jersey Child and Adolescent Psychiatry for years. She successfully integrates nutrition and functional medicine into the treatment of her patients. In 2013, she opened a gourmet restaurant, Ancient Grains Fresh Pasta, in Brooklyn, New York. She co-authored the "Sicilian Secret Diet Plan," a book with her husband, Giovanni Campanile, MD. Together, they have formulated a Mediterranean diet supplement, *Healthy to 100*, which provides most of the essential nutrients in the Mediterranean Diet. Both are available on Amazon. Sandra hosts a popular podcast with her husband, "The Sicilian Secret Diet" which can be heard on Spotify, Apple Podcast and Castbox.

Connect with Sandra:

Office phone for appointments (in-person and virtual): (973)618-0100

Website: siciliansecret.com

Instagram, Facebook, You Tube, Tik Tok: @siciliansecretdiet

CHAPTER 9

SEEDS OF TOMORROW

PLANNING FOR A HEALTHY PREGNANCY AND BEYOND

Adria Rothfeld, DC, MS, CNS

MY STORY

I was determined to prevent history from repeating itself, but my plan backfired spectacularly.

Our family spent summers in upstate New York, where I was often drowsy from Benadryl since the trees and grass were my kryptonite. I ruined many Mah Jong nights for my mom, as my eczema always seemed to flare up on those occasions. Mah Jong was a decadent affair, where Mom went all out on junk food reserved for the players, but as kids, we found loopholes, allowing me to stuff myself with candy and soda. I had asthma, a constant belly ache, and was the skinniest girl in my class. Clearly, I was a hugely allergic kid with a significant immune imbalance.

Back then, most people, including physicians, knew very little about how prenatal lifestyle factors could influence their offspring. I was determined to do things right when it came time for me to get pregnant. I read the scarce books available 30 years ago. I had a complete medical workup (which was anything but) and was told, "Your labs are fine; go for it." I avoided shellfish for fear of hepatitis, abstained from alcohol, and didn't take any prescription medications, so I followed the basic rules.

I craved smoked salmon (likely due to an omega-3 fatty acid deficiency) and ate it often, nitrates and farm-raised PCBs galore. I developed a rash in the corner of my mouth (suggestive of B vitamin deficiencies), and my eczema returned with a vengeance. I took a prenatal tablet that could've choked a horse, with so much iron that I gave birth to an eight-pound nine-ounce baby and what felt like a two-pound hemorrhoid. While my prenatal contained plenty of folic acid, I later discovered I have a potent MTHFR gene variant, which discourages the use of folic acid in favor of an appropriate methylated form.

On my due date, mistakenly thought to be a harbinger of smooth sailing to come, I gave birth to a healthy baby boy (and the hemorrhoid). Unfortunately, things began to derail soon after. My son developed an award-winning, sleep-depriving case of colic that lasted over a year. He inherited my eczema and was sensitive to most soaps, detergents, and foods, etc. He seemed to puke more breastmilk than he drank, but I persisted, fearing how he'd react to solid foods. Croup started at eight months and recurred with every mild respiratory infection. Sensory integration issues turned baths and haircuts into harrowing experiences, and tags on his clothing would trigger meltdowns.

As a functional medicine practitioner, I struggled to understand how we ended up in this situation. I realized it was time for an *even deeper dive* to help not only my son and myself but also break this cycle for my future children and, hopefully, generations to come. Years of targeted research and clinical experience brought me to this point. Never has the phrase, "necessity is the *mother* of invention," rung truer.

For my family (and many of my patients), there are genetics that aren't working in our favor. However, most of these genetic variants aren't written in stone; they largely depend upon the influence of environmental factors.

THE SKILL

This chapter will outline proven methods to support the most favorable circumstances before and during pregnancy, arming you with the greatest advantages for fertility and the well-being of your family.

Egg and Sperm: To say our girls are picky would be an understatement. Only one sperm is chosen for the lead role, and that winner is nothing short of an Olympic gold medalist. Each ejaculation contains between 80-300 million sperm, but only a few hundred reach the egg, and only one grand champion is selected to fertilize it. Now that's a competition!

Unlike a female's eggs, which are present from about 20 weeks gestation until menopause, sperm develop over a 70-day period. The health of sperm largely depends upon the male's lifestyle during that time. Sperm health impacts not only pregnancy outcomes but also has 'epigenetic' effects, meaning that sperm quality can influence whether genes turn on or off in the baby and can impact future disease risk.

Sadly, the news about sperm isn't encouraging; thirty percent of infertility cases are due to unhealthy sperm. A sobering meta-analysis of 185 studies involving over 40,000 men found that the average sperm count dropped 59% between 1973 and 2011.

We must therefore consider these two to three months as 'sperm boot camp' and adopt proven lifestyle behaviors that can have generational impacts. Sperm health reflects the overall health of the father. Unhealthy sperm indicates that developing cells are unable to mature normally, serving as a wake-up call on many levels.

Oxidative Stress: An arch enemy of sperm is oxidative stress, proven to be the main cause of male infertility. While oxidative stress may seem like an abstract concept, it boils down to the fact that while we need oxygen to survive, an imbalance between oxidants (free radicals) and antioxidants, which favor the former, can wreak havoc on our bodies.

Oxidative stress can also impact ovarian egg quantity and quality. Research suggests that a contributor to unexplained infertility, which affects 15% of couples in the US, is linked to oxidative stress.

Endocrine Disruptors: Key contributors to oxidative stress include exposure to endocrine (hormone) disrupting chemicals. An extensive five-year review examined the impact of BPA (present in plastic water bottles, canned goods, coated paper products, dental sealants, and much more) as well as air pollution, pesticides, heavy metals (mercury/arsenic/cadmium), parabens (personal care products, some medications, even foods), on male and female fertility.

In women, BPA disrupts menstrual cycles and is linked to PCOS, fibroids, endometriosis, preterm birth, and increased miscarriage rates. In men, exposure impairs sperm quantity and quality as well as libido. The study concluded that many environmental contaminants were associated with reduced fertility in men and women.

Other contributors to oxidative stress include cigarette smoke, recreational drug use, alcohol, exposure to radiation, high-sugar diets, other non-BPA plastics, infections, obesity, malnutrition, and iron overload. Maternal nicotine exposure (whether through active or passive smoking) is associated with multiple pregnancy complications, including miscarriage. Alcohol use during pregnancy is linked to low-birth-weight infants and increased risks of pregnancy loss and congenital abnormalities.

Caffeine: In men, caffeine seems to have no significant effect on sperm, but soda and other soft drinks can have a negative impact. In women, caffeine can lead to lower birth weight infants, and moderate to heavy consumption (over 150 mg/day) significantly increases the risk of miscarriages in the first and second trimesters. Even light caffeine use (under 150 mg/day) can heighten miscarriage risk for those with a history of prior miscarriages.

I know I sound like Debbie Downer, and this information is not only frightening but also depressing. The good news is that many of these exposures can be mitigated through actionable lifestyle modifications. The key is to tip the scales to favor antioxidants over free radicals and clean alternatives vs. toxic ones. **Studies have shown that simply swapping one serving of conventional fruits or vegetables for organic options each day significantly improves sperm quality and quantity while reducing pregnancy loss.** The lowest sperm counts were in men with the highest pesticide levels.

It's not difficult to replace plastic water bottles with stainless steel or glass, use non-toxic beauty and household products, avoid high-mercury seafood (what is this obsession with sushi anyway?), limit pesticide/chemical exposures by using non-toxic alternatives for lawn care and insect control, and make lifestyle changes regarding smoking, alcohol and recreational drugs.

The liver and gut microbiome neutralize these toxins and pollutants. If the liver is overwhelmed with endocrine disruptors and other chemicals, detoxification capacity is likely to be impaired.

Regarding the Gut Microbiome and Probiotics: The first 1,000 days of life (from conception to age two) is when the gut microbiota (microbes colonizing the GI tract) is established. Therefore, these first two years provide a critical window of opportunity for intervention. Early dysbiosis (imbalanced bacterial flora) is linked to immune dysfunction, including allergic diseases, colic, and even obesity.

Research has shown that administering probiotics (foods or supplements that contain live microorganisms intended to maintain levels of good bacteria) and prebiotics (high-fiber foods that feed beneficial bacteria), both pre and postnatally, is a safe and effective way to improve pregnancy outcomes and the health of the offspring. Probiotic supplements during pregnancy and infancy can reduce the incidence of food allergies and eczema, especially in children at high risk of allergic sensitization. *I wish someone had told me that 30 years ago so I could have gotten some sleep!*

Low levels of beneficial bacteria in infants (associated with C-sections, preterm birth, early antibiotic exposure, and low birth weight) are linked to future prevalence of obesity, diabetes, and metabolic disorders. Using probiotics pre and postnatally to prevent and/or repair any associated early dysbiosis is a viable treatment option.

In addition to probiotic supplementation, a diverse intake of fruits, vegetables and fiber sources, fermented foods, sleep, exercise, outdoor activities, and interaction with pets can help support a healthy microbiome.

Fats: Essential fatty acids are fats that the body cannot produce, making it *essential* to consume them through diet and/or supplements.

The brain is 60% fat, and a baby's developing brain relies on essential fatty acids for healthy development. The omega-3 fatty acid DHA is concentrated in brain and retinal tissues and is most critically needed during the 3rd trimester through 18 months after birth. Food sources include seafood, dairy, and egg yolks. Supplementing during pregnancy and ensuring that the baby receives DHA through breast milk or enriched formula is recommended.

It is crucial for moms to incorporate a variety of dietary fats such as fish oils, chia and flax seeds, olive oil, avocado oil, and nut oils. Arachidonic acid, found in butter, egg yolks, grass-fed meat, and shellfish, is important for fetal brain growth and development but can promote inflammation in excess, especially in women with endometriosis and pelvic pain.

The key is balance. Essential fatty acids ultimately form chemicals called prostaglandins, which help regulate the inflammatory response. Partially hydrogenated fats, found in many processed baked goods, snacks, fried foods, margarine, and coffee creamers, promote highly inflammatory prostaglandins.

Prostaglandin imbalances are linked to pelvic pain and cramping, mood changes, and premenstrual fluid retention associated with PMS and endometriosis. Endometriosis accounts for 15% of infertility in women and affects 6-10% of the female population.

Body Composition: Over 40% of reproductive-aged men and women in the U.S. are obese. Obese women generally take longer to conceive and face higher risks of miscarriage, C-sections, gestational diabetes, preeclampsia, and PCOS.

Normalizing weight—both under (BMI < 18.5) and overweight (BMI > 25)—can resolve fertility issues in up to 15% of cases. For individuals who are overweight, losing ten pounds can dramatically impact fertility. Insufficient body fat can adversely impact hormones and impair ovulation.

In men, obesity not only impairs fertility, but sperm from obese males can worsen IVF outcomes. Body fat is also where we store most of our toxins.

Exercise: Moderate exercise can help restore fertility by supporting a healthier BMI. Exercise improves ovulation, reduces insulin resistance, and leads to weight loss in women with PCOS.

However, exercise can be a double-edged sword. Studies have shown that overtraining can reduce ovulation in women, particularly for those who train vigorously for more than sixty minutes/day. In men, overtraining can reduce sperm quality. Thirty to sixty minutes/day of moderate daily exercise reduces risk unless it's overly strenuous or leads to low BMI. If you have trouble recovering (not getting stronger or faster), these can be signs of overtraining.

While sedentary lifestyles aren't recommended, overtraining, low body fat, and insufficient dietary fat can create a perfect storm for infertility. If the body feels strained, it will divert calories away from reproductive pathways. Being underweight can lead to inadequate nutrition, adversely affecting fetal growth and resulting in low-birth-weight infants.

I've been discussing complex topics, but the single most important lifestyle factor for a healthy pregnancy, delivery, and baby is improving body composition. This is where diet comes into play, and a healthy diet for improving antioxidant status, blood sugar regulation, and inflammation aligns considerably with one for optimizing body composition.

I've talked about epigenetic effects related to sperm health, but numerous studies show that maternal nutritional status can permanently alter the developing fetus's epigenome, consequently impacting long-term health.

Dietary factors that negatively impact fertility and contribute to obesity include high intakes of red and processed meat, potatoes, full-fat dairy, sugary drinks, high saturated fats as well as trans fatty acids, and refined carbohydrates. These should be replaced with high-fiber whole grains, seafood, nuts, seeds, fruits, vegetables, lean dairy, poultry, unprocessed meat, and essential fatty acids from EPA/DHA, flax, and olive oil.

While much of the research focuses on fertility, there is significant overlap with maternal diet during pregnancy concerning pregnancy outcomes and the health of the baby. The dietary recommendations mentioned above are *essentially identical* in their favorable effects on multiple parameters. Incorporating these foods can help reduce inflammation and support blood sugar regulation, both linked to reducing numerous pregnancy-related complications.

Foods and Supplements: Foods and supplements rich in vitamins C, E, D, folate, glutathione, selenium, zinc, omega-3 EPA/DHA, CoQ10, luteolin, lycopene, and carnitine favorably impact sperm quality and male fertility. For female fertility, similar findings apply; folate, B vitamins, trace minerals, and antioxidants like vitamins C and E, glutathione, CoQ10, as well as EPA/DHA, and vitamin D were supportive.

Folate deserves special mention. Every prenatal I have examined contains some form of folate since it is well-established that this vitamin is crucial for reducing the risk of birth defects in the brain and spinal cord. However, 60% of the population has a genetic variant known as MTHFR. Those with MTHFR are advised to supplement with a methylated form of folate (5-MTHF or folinic) instead of folic acid since those with the gene mutation struggle to convert synthetic folic acid into its active form.

Research has shown that couples undergoing IVF who switch from folic acid to the 5-MTHF form of folate experience increased conception rates. A study published in the Journal of Assisted Reproductive Technology concluded that: "regular doses of folic acid should be abandoned in the presence of MTHFR mutations as the genetic background of the patient precluded a correct supply of the active compound."

EMF Exposure: Keep those laptops and phones away from the family jewels. This means no phones in pockets and keeping the laptop off laps. This can help reduce the EMF-associated oxidative stress that negatively impacts sperm quality.

Thyroid Dysfunction: Even functional hypothyroidism, where lab results still fall within conventional levels, can lead to infertility. In men, hypothyroidism affects sperm quality, quantity, motility, and libido. It's crucial to measure thyroid hormone levels and antibodies before and during pregnancy.

Unadapted Stress: Lack of healthy coping skills and support can impact fertility. Various hormonal downstream effects from this type of stress can affect ovulation and sperm production. Couples undergoing IVF/IUI who had more supportive nurses/doctors and access to counseling services reported better pregnancy outcomes. Exercise has also proven effective for improving mood during pregnancy.

Other Factors: Tight underwear can impair sperm formation. Switching from typical daytime underwear to boxers (or none) for bed has been shown to improve sperm quality. The same goes for hot tubs with regard to damaging sperm.

Breastfeeding: Pregnancy involves an essential but dramatic shift in the mother's physiology. The immune system becomes hyper-vigilant, but this is normal. The microbiome of a pregnant woman resembles that of an obese one, again, perfectly normal. After childbirth, hormonal shifts can adversely affect insulin resistance, sugar cravings, mood, sleep disturbances, and immune dysfunction. *Breast milk to the rescue!* The hormones it releases in mom help reshape the microbiome, immune system, and the insulin response back to the pre-pregnant state.

Breast milk contains growth factors that optimize immunity, inflammation, blood sugar regulation, and nervous system function in infants. It also helps modulate the infant's early gut microbiome, a promising tool for allergy prevention. The health of the baby is closely tied to the mother's diet, which impacts the health of the infant's microbiome.

My goal for this chapter was to provide a roadmap for couples, with actionable steps, emphasizing that this is the time to be all in regarding adopting healthy lifestyle habits. Remember, you have nine months to build your new person, and your actions during this time are proven to significantly impact your child well into adulthood.

CHECKLIST INCORPORATING MANY OF THE CONCEPTS OUTLINED IN THIS CHAPTER:

- Men: Clean up your act, especially two to three months before planning to conceive.

- Reduce toxin exposure: Use stainless or glass water bottles with filtered water.

- Avoid high-mercury seafood.

- Eat organic food whenever possible; even just one serving/day can make a significant impact.

- Don't smoke, and limit caffeine.

- Incorporate a variety of fats: Omega-3 (seafood, fish oils, flax, chia), olive oil, avocado, and nut oils, and in moderation, egg yolks, grass-fed beef, and butter.

- Consume antioxidant-rich foods: fruits, vegetables, herbs, spices, beans, nuts, seeds, and fermented foods.

- Keep cell phones and laptops out of pockets and off laps.

- Check thyroid labs, including thyroid antibodies.

- Choose a prenatal with methylated folate or folinic instead of folic acid.

- Ensure time for fun, relaxation, and activities that bring you joy to minimize stress.

- Men: Don't wear tight underwear to bed.

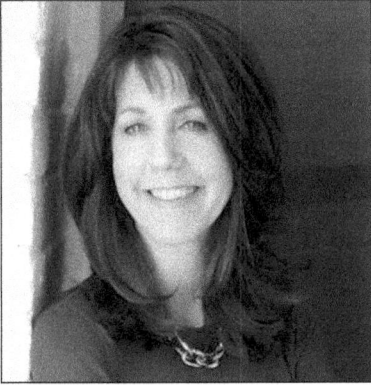

Dr. Adria Rothfeld, DC, MS, CNS, a chiropractic physician, graduated summa cum laude from Palmer College of Chiropractic. After building a successful family practice with her husband, Dr. Lee Magenheim, Dr. Adria realized she needed to broaden her knowledge to provide comprehensive care. Many patients were pain-free but inquired about more personalized approaches for various health challenges. They were disenchanted with allopathic rushed office visits, cursory lab testing, and an illness-focused healthcare model.

Dr. Adria earned a Master's in Human Nutrition and became a Certified Nutrition Specialist, requiring advanced studies and rigorous examination. She's completed all the Institute for Functional Medicine training modules and attended numerous courses focusing on holistic, root-cause approaches. However, she acknowledges her best lessons come from listening to her patients—her best teachers.

Her passion intensified when her son Jake presented as an infant with colic, eczema, and sensory integration issues. Inspired by her own childhood medical history, she was determined not to allow history to repeat itself. Turning again to integrative medicine, she helped her son overcome many challenges she faced as a child and became an advocate for current and prospective parents.

Dr. Adria's patients value the time she dedicates to assessing their individual needs. She creates truly personalized programs for a variety of health concerns centered on education and lifestyle modifications.

This chapter is dedicated to building a solid foundation for pregnancy, promoting the healthiest environment for fertility, and the well-being of parents and their children.

Dr. Adria resides in New Jersey on a horse farm with her husband, two horses, Cody and Hazel, and several rescue cats. In her free time, she enjoys the outdoors, riding, cooking, reading, exercising, and spending time with her family.

Connect with Dr. Adria:

Websites: www.thenutritionalwellnesscenter.com
www.doctoradria.com

Instagram: @dradriarothfeld

Facebook: https://www.facebook.com/TheNutritionalWellnessCenter

ENVIRONMENTAL EXPOSURES

*"Our health is intertwined with the health of our environment.
Toxins not only threaten the natural world
but also jeopardize our own well-being."*

~ Dr. Florence Williams

ENVIRONMENTAL EXPOSURES: AN OVERVIEW

The Environmental Pillar represents both *the power of nature* and *navigation against the many health threats we face* as we live our lives.

I think of it in terms of key concepts that are essential to understand. In the coming chapters (and also in some previous ones) you'll find some highlights with very valuable, practical, and unique insights.

A. Utilizing the Power of Nature

Nature is powerful. Earth has been created with all that we inherently need: sunlight, fresh air, water, plants, and energy.

B. Barriers

Our bodies have been designed with "barriers" protecting us from invaders. We have them on our skin, our brain, and wherever our body is connected to the outside, for example, at the intestinal lining and the airways. Protecting and nourishing these barriers enhances our immune defenses and lowers the risk of pathogens, like bacteria, and risky substances from entering our circulation.

C. Reducing Our Burden of Environmental Toxins-Pollution

Three Essential Concepts:

The Precautionary Principle.

Did you know that it often takes years to decades to establish clear links between exposure to a substance and health harms? *This is a delay in proving harm!* In healthcare, we've seen it with things that used to be glorified but now have become or are becoming taboo with proven harm—cigarettes, asbestos, lead, the pesticide DDT, Teflon, and many more. It's to our greatest benefit, when there is an emerging concern about something, to take notice and start proactively avoiding it when you can, substitute it for better alternatives, and make an effort to continue to stay aware.

Avoid—Include—Remove (A.I.R).

We come into contact daily with environmental pollutants in our air (indoor and outdoor), water, food, personal care products, and through things like radiation. We're also surrounded by psychological toxicity in the news, on social media, and in our community. Our bodies only have the capacity to deal with a certain amount at a time until they become overwhelmed.

That's why *avoiding* them when you can is so important. Simple, thoughtful strategies, several of which you'll learn about within this book, can help lighten the load on your body.

In addition to avoiding exposures when we can, it's paramount to support our body's inherent ways of detoxifying—*getting rid of* these pollutants and toxins from inside ourselves.

The team leaders of our "clean-up crew" are the:

- Liver, which is the powerhouse of preparing and packaging the products for removal (i.e., through urine, bowel movements, and sweat)

- Kidneys via urine (which is why you want to stay hydrated)

- Digestive tract via bowel movements (which is why you want to avoid constipation)

- Skin via sweat (which is why saunas can potentially have benefits in addition to sweating during exercise)

- Lungs via deep diaphragmatic breaths (which help to pump lymphatic fluid)

- Microbiome (plays an integral role in many ways)

- Lymphatic system, which is our filter and sewage system that keeps things flowing on their way out

- Glymphatic system - the brain's lymphatic system - which gets activated when we sleep

We can support these by *including* these foundations:

- Providing strategically supportive nutrients
- Staying hydrated
- Strategies for avoiding constipation
- Moving in ways that support lymphatic flow
- Keeping our resilience to the world around us with meaningful connections, nurturing inner wisdom and self-regulation.

Make your home a safe haven.

Home is the one place we have the most control. It's where we can implement our values most effectively. Help reduce the pollution by leaving your shoes at the door, swapping out cleaning and self-care products, keeping quality food in your pantry, purifying your air and water, choosing what you watch and listen to, and anything else that you find hard to do when you're out in the world. The benefits become exponential!

CHAPTER 10

THE RHYTHM OF THE SUN

USING LIGHT FOR MOOD, METABOLISM, AND MORE

Laurel Parker-Chan

As above, so below...

MY STORY

When I woke up from surgery, I felt like I was free-falling.

A wave of panic swept over me, so powerful it felt like drowning. The room was spinning, but I was still. I had gone in for a routine procedure, something that was supposed to be "simple." Instead, I woke up feeling like I had been hurled backward, to a place I thought I'd left behind. Suddenly, the years of healing, of building my strength, felt as fragile as glass.

Just days before, I was a healthy, vibrant 21-year-old, fully immersed in health and wellness. I had a thriving business, years of experience as a gymnastics coach, and a firm foundation in biochemistry and biophysics. But now, nothing seemed to matter. This mental darkness felt relentless. I could hardly believe that a physical procedure had shaken me so deeply, so completely.

Complex PTSD had been a part of my life since I first went to a therapist at 18. But by 2021, I had been in such a beautiful, peaceful place—mentally, emotionally, spiritually. I had found a therapist who had helped me use somatic practices to reconnect with myself, and I thought I'd found a steady, lasting peace. But this surgery, and whatever it stirred up in me, took me back to square one. For weeks afterward, I felt paralyzed by fear, sadness, and a darkness I couldn't explain.

I needed a way out, something that went beyond conventional health practices. I was desperate for light in every sense of the word. And in a moment of sheer determination, I dove into researching everything that could explain and possibly heal this state. This journey led me somewhere unexpected: applied quantum biology and circadian health. I discovered that natural light could actually impact my mental health, mood, and even the biochemistry of my body. It was the missing piece, something I hadn't fully grasped until I felt its effects in my own life.

BUILDING MY FOUNDATION

Before that fateful surgery, my life was built on a foundation of health and wellness that felt as solid as bedrock. My upbringing was a unique blend of influences, shaping me in ways I am only now beginning to fully understand. My father, who grew up in Hong Kong, believed that health was a lifelong journey, one that demanded intention and resilience. He'd often remind me, "Nothing is easy, especially the good stuff in life."

He'd bring these principles to life in practical, sometimes challenging ways—like the bitter herbal teas he would have me drink at different times of the year, carefully crafted to prepare our bodies for each season. It didn't matter that they tasted terrible. He'd tell me that these tonics were part of honoring the natural cycles and respecting what each season asked of us. Health, he taught me, was an investment in my future self, a form of discipline and gratitude.

My mother, however, brought a much more complicated layer to my journey. She had her own health struggles when she was younger and relied on alternative health practices to turn things around. Because of her, we were raised on herbal tonics she made herself, brews that seemed strange and mysterious to me as a child. I can still picture her mixing ingredients and doling out bitter, earthy drinks for us to sip, insisting they were essential for our health. I thought of them as "witch's brews," partly because of their taste and partly because her presence felt intense, almost otherworldly.

But my mother's influence wasn't just about health; it cast a shadow over much of my childhood. She left when I was only nine, leaving my father and me to care for my seven siblings, the youngest only in first grade. When she eventually returned, she brought with her a new man and made it clear that her presence was out of obligation, not love. She would drive me to gymnastics practice, make sure we kept the garden, and enforce her ideas about life and health, but her presence was as distant as it was disruptive.

Her views on health and education were equally rigid and often at odds with my own curiosity. She was deeply distrustful of organized education, convinced that traditional schooling was a form of indoctrination. I only began to understand her perspective much later, but it created a rift between us much before then. When I announced in 2017 that I was going to Rensselaer Polytechnic Institute (RPI) to study biochemistry and biophysics, she was furious, believing that I was abandoning my roots for a "mainstream" education. We haven't spoken since.

As painful as that experience was, I recognize now that some of her warnings weren't entirely unfounded—at least when it came to the biases in mainstream health and education. But beyond that, her words left wounds that took me years to confront. She would belittle me for being a "try hard," criticize me for excelling academically, and remind me constantly of how different we were as one of the only Asian-American families in our small town. Her words and the absence she left in our family became a weight I carried, one that I have come to see as the result of her own unhealed trauma.

In the end, her complex legacy is part of what pushed me to seek answers for myself, to dive deeply into the sciences and challenge the perspectives I'd been given. And despite the painful memories, I know that part of my resilience, my drive to understand health and healing, is rooted in the challenges she set before me.

THE TURNING POINT: THE DISCOVERY OF THE CYSTS

When I went in for a routine check-up at the gynecologist, I didn't expect anything out of the ordinary. So, hearing that I had not one but two ovarian cysts was a shock, though my doctors assured me it was nothing serious. One was the size of a grapefruit, the other a lemon. They advised a simple surgery to remove them, and I was told it would be straightforward, almost routine. With my foundation in health, I felt confident I could handle this—both the procedure and the recovery.

But what I wasn't prepared for was the mental and emotional upheaval that would follow. When I woke up from surgery, that confidence was gone. Instead of feeling relieved, I was enveloped in a consuming sense of dread. It wasn't like waking up from anesthesia; it was like waking up to a nightmare. It felt as if all the progress I'd made in healing my mental health, in finding balance, had vanished. The physical trauma of the surgery triggered an emotional flood that pulled me under.

In the days that followed, it was as if each sunrise brought with it a fresh wave of darkness as if the familiar rhythm of day and night had somehow been thrown off course. I had experienced dark days before, but this felt different. There were mornings when I could hardly bring myself to get out of bed, even as I could hear birds outside my window or see the light starting to change in the sky. It was as if something vital, some essential connection to myself, had been severed. The old methods of self-care and grounding I'd relied on seemed useless, and it scared me.

This darkness clouded every corner of my life, casting shadows over the dreams I'd worked so hard to build. I was terrified and struggling to hold on, wondering if I'd ever get back to where I was before. I knew that in order to find peace again, I would need something different, something powerful enough to pull me back to the light.

A LIGHT IN THE DARKNESS: DISCOVERING CIRCADIAN HEALTH

Desperate for answers, I turned to what I knew best—research and the pursuit of knowledge. I stumbled across applied quantum biology, a science that explores the subtle yet profound ways our bodies respond to natural forces. Within that realm, I discovered circadian health and the role of sunlight in regulating the body's internal rhythms.

I learned that our bodies are wired to respond to the natural cycle of day and night. Sunlight, particularly in the morning, signals the release of hormones that wake us up, energize us, and set the pace for our metabolism and mood throughout the day. And at night, in the absence of light, our bodies naturally wind down, preparing us for rest.

The more I read, the more I felt like I'd stumbled onto something sacred. This was health in its most elemental form, health rooted in the rhythms of nature. And as I began incorporating sunlight into my daily routine, I could feel my body recalibrating, my mind finding calm in ways it hadn't before. Slowly, I felt myself healing, reconnecting with that peace I'd lost.

THE SKILL

Most of us understand that our bodies need essential nutrients like magnesium, vitamin D, and protein to function well. But one nutrient often goes overlooked, even though it's freely available every day: light. Much more than something that brightens our world, light is a key player in our biology. It fuels processes as essential as hormone production, metabolism, and emotional balance. When we begin to view light as a nutrient, it shifts our habits, helping us become more intentional in connecting with the sun's energy.

Just like with any other health practice, getting the right "dose" of light requires awareness and skill. A great way to start is by simply observing how much time you spend in natural light throughout the day. For many people, sunlight exposure can be surprisingly limited due to time spent indoors or artificial lighting that lacks the full spectrum our bodies need.

To support this awareness, I often suggest an app called MyCircadianApp by Sarah Kleiner Wellness. This tool can guide you in understanding how much time you spend in naturally lit environments, helping you track the light levels of your surroundings and even providing insights on the timing and strength of UVB rays throughout the day. Knowing when UVB is available is key for vitamin D production, especially if you live in areas where sunlight can be limited by season. With MyCircadianApp, you can log your time spent outside and monitor the brightness of your environment, making it easier to see where you can incorporate more natural light exposure.

THE SCIENCE OF LIGHT AS A NUTRIENT: UVA AND THE POMC PATHWAY

The effects of natural light extend well beyond what we see. Each morning, shortly after sunrise, the rising levels of UVA light kick off a powerful metabolic pathway known as the POMC (Pro-opiomelanocortin) pathway. This pathway is foundational for health because it sits upstream of several other important processes, including appetite regulation, immune response, and energy metabolism. By simply getting outside for a few minutes of morning sunlight, we're able to stimulate this pathway naturally, setting our bodies up for balanced hormone production and metabolic health.

Studies show that natural sunlight, especially UVA and UVB, can trigger hormone releases that artificial light cannot fully replicate. These exposures signal our body's release of beta-endorphins (boosting mood) and serotonin (supporting sleep and emotional balance). When we miss out on these cues from natural light, our POMC pathway doesn't function as well, and over time, this can affect mood, energy levels, and even our relationship with food.

LIGHT AS AN EMF: WHY NATURAL LIGHT MATTERS

Understanding light as a nutrient involves recognizing it as a type of electromagnetic frequency (EMF), one that interacts directly with our cells. While artificial light sources—like LEDs or screens—provide light, they often miss the broad spectrum that natural sunlight offers. This broad spectrum is rich in wavelengths our bodies recognize and thrive on, from UVA and UVB to infrared and red light, which support everything from tissue repair to energy production at a cellular level.

The challenge with artificial lighting and windows is that they filter out many of these wavelengths. Glass, plastic, and other barriers can block certain types of light, meaning that even sitting by a window doesn't give you the full range of light's benefits. For this reason, stepping outside—even for a short break—is the most effective way to receive the broad-spectrum light our bodies need. Think of it as a "multi-vitamin" of light, essential for your body's daily requirements.

MODERN LIFE AND BLUE LIGHT: PROTECTING OUR DOPAMINE PATHWAYS

While natural light nourishes us, artificial light—particularly blue light from screens and LED lighting—can be a source of stress on our bodies. Blue light, which is abundant in most screens and newer technology, stimulates our dopamine pathways. Dopamine is the neurotransmitter responsible for pleasure, motivation, and reward, but when it's constantly overstimulated by artificial blue light, it can become dysregulated. This dysregulation contributes to our dependence on screens and can even fuel feelings of anxiety and cravings for the constant "reward" that tech provides. (https://academic.oup.com/endo/article/159/5/1992/4931051)

Excessive blue light, especially later in the day, disrupts our natural circadian rhythm, making it harder for us to feel tired at night and more alert during the day. One simple solution is to make sure you're prioritizing natural light exposure during the day, as natural sunlight has the balanced spectrum our bodies need to counteract the effects of artificial light. Using blue-light-blocking glasses or software filters can also help reduce exposure, particularly in the evening.

GETTING STARTED WITH LIGHT AS A NUTRIENT: PRACTICAL TIPS

1. Track and Adjust Your Daily Light Exposure: Begin each day by noting how much natural light exposure you're getting. MyCircadianApp can help you see patterns and find more opportunities to step outside, even if it's just a few minutes in the morning and at midday.

2. Prioritize Morning Sunlight: Start your day by stepping outside during sunrise or early morning. This is when UVA light is most beneficial, signaling your POMC pathway to initiate important metabolic processes that keep energy and mood balanced.

3. Limit Screen Time, Especially After Sunset: Be mindful of screen use in the evening, as blue light disrupts melatonin production, a hormone essential for restful sleep. Blue-light-blocking tools can help, but ideally, winding down with minimal artificial light is best.

4. Take Short Outdoor Breaks: Step outside whenever possible, even if it's just for a few minutes. Remember, natural sunlight offers a full spectrum of wavelengths that supports everything from cellular health to mental clarity.

5. Use Blue-Light-Blocking Glasses When Needed: If your work requires long hours on screens, consider wearing tinted blue-light-blocking glasses during the day, especially toward the evening, to protect your dopamine and circadian cycles. These can be even more essential if you're exposed to screens before bed.

6. Optimize Indoor Lighting for Circadian Health: Create a circadian-friendly environment by using incandescent or full-spectrum amber LED bulbs, especially in rooms where you spend your mornings and evenings. Red or amber night lights can be especially helpful for kids' rooms and hallways, offering safety and calming light that doesn't interfere with sleep cycles.

7. Position Your Workspace Near a Window and Open It When Possible: Facing a window helps your brain distinguish between artificial and natural light, helping it stay calibrated to the day-night cycle. Cracking the window, even slightly, lets a fuller spectrum of natural light filter in, benefiting your body even when you're indoors.

FINDING BALANCE IN SUN EXPOSURE

While sunlight is a powerful and natural way to enhance health, finding balance is essential to avoid overexposure. Our bodies offer somatic feedback, like feeling extreme warmth or discomfort after prolonged sun exposure, but it's still wise to integrate sunlight slowly, like any new health habit. Begin with gentle, shorter exposures, and build gradually as you listen to your body's responses.

If you're new to light therapy or don't have the time to study its complexities, working with a professional well-versed in safe sun exposure can be invaluable. Light therapy has nuances, and overexposure can have serious consequences, as many of us are aware—most notably, skin cancer risk. A professional can guide you through a tailored approach that helps you balance sunlight's health benefits while prioritizing skin safety.

By treating light as a vital nutrient, you're already taking the first step toward realigning your body with the natural rhythms that sustain us. Just small, consistent efforts to expose yourself to natural light, limit artificial light, and prioritize the sunlight we're meant to experience can lead to profound shifts in your health and mindset.

And yet, this is just the beginning. If you're intrigued by the power of nature to heal and energize, reach out to me to explore further. Whether it's a class or a one-on-one coaching session, we'll go deeper into optimizing your light exposure and using the rhythms of nature to transform your health journey. Together, we'll uncover the next steps to harnessing light as a foundation for lifelong, limitless wellness.

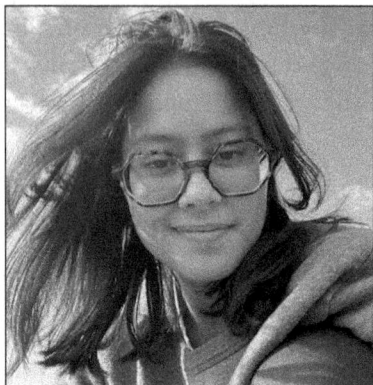

Laurel Parker-Chan is the founder and CEO of Limitless Wellness LLC, a health consultancy dedicated to empowering clients with natural, science-backed approaches to wellness. Educated both in and beyond the classrooms of Rensselaer Polytechnic Institute, where she studied biochemistry and biophysics, Laurel has been mentored by world-renowned experts and has gained deep insights through years of consistent work with clients. Her entrepreneurial journey includes certifications from Cornell University, hands-on experience with Human Garage, and training with Health Optimization Medicine & Practice.

With a unique blend of traditional education, advanced certifications, and holistic health philosophies, Laurel teaches clients how to harness the natural elements—light, nutrition, movement, and more—to build sustainable health. Her approach draws from both science and lived experience, aiming to help others achieve self-sovereignty in their health. Today, she spends much of her time giving back to the community, offering free classes and one-on-one coaching sessions that share the fundamentals of wellness.

An outdoor enthusiast, Laurel loves hiking waterfalls with her Siberian husky. You won't find her on mainstream social media, as she believes in a more direct, decentralized connection. For inquiries or to learn about upcoming classes, reach out directly to see how she's redefining health from the inside out.

Connect with Laurel:

Email: thelimitlesswellness@gmail.com

LinkTree: https://linktr.ee/limitlesslaurel

CHAPTER 11

A PRESCRIPTION TO BLOOM

HOW TO RECLAIM YOUR HEALTH WITH HERBS

Elina K. Restrepo, RPh, ND, CNC

MY STORY

"I'm sorry, you have six months, maybe nine. I wish there were more I could do." His death sentence was off by 13 years.

What started as a very personal endeavor became my life's mission. My father was diagnosed with cancer while I was still a young and curious student in pharmacy school. The outlook was grim, and conventional medical therapies were limited due to the late-stage findings. Post-treatment, he would inevitably be reduced to another statistic befitting the diagnosis. Immediately, we arranged a meeting with a top oncologist. Walking into the unknown with our hopes high, we settled onto a couch in a dim corner. Thirty minutes later, we were called into the lion's den. That's when I heard, "I'm sorry…" and just like that, those two little words packed enough power to shatter us.

Emotionless, he offered a hamster wheel of prescriptions, starting with one for depression, one for anxiety, a sleeping pill, and another for pain. After throwing me a forced smile, my father graciously said, "No, thank you." My heart pumped out of my chest, clenching my jaw. *Are you freaking kidding me?* I thought. *The chief of a highly regarded department at a very prestigious hospital in one of the biggest cities in the world just gave us a timeline.*

As we stood up, I felt my knees buckle. I took the deepest, longest, most excruciating breath I'd ever taken. Devastated, we walked out in silence, our heads hung low. We avoided making eye contact, and with pits in our stomachs, we made our way down to the parking garage.

My father was a gifted and passionate musician with a real zest for life. He was intelligent, spiritual, humble, kind, and deeply compassionate. I was lucky to have him set the standard for me of what a genuinely good individual should be. He was my hero. He raised his two children with the same core values, although his mouthy Brooklyn-bred daughter occasionally needed to vocalize her opinions. Needless to say, I had unfinished business. I let my parents out of the elevator on the ground level and shot back up to the fourth floor. To kick someone while they're down is the absolute lowest thing you can do in my book. I felt it my duty to strip him of his Godliness before I turned my back and walked out the door. *He will never forget me.*

Realizing I had to take matters into my own hands, I began to feel the world's weight on my shoulders. I was about to lose my father, and I wasn't ready for that reality. Is anyone ever? My days at the library turned into nights and late nights into early mornings engulfed in reading all I could find on ailing bodies. Completely absorbed, I ignored a sign from the universe that placed the self-help section across my desk. It all caught up to me shortly before graduation. I wasn't sleeping because I was too afraid of wasting time. I barely ate, living off of the vending machine nearby. I ran on caffeine and adrenaline. Burning a candle at both ends, I was exhausted mentally and physically.

After studying most of the required textbooks for medical students, I tried to wrap my head around the fact that 5000 pages offered close to zero on nutrition, no mention of the mind-body connection, and nothing on true healing. It was all about cutting, discarding, and prescribing to treat symptoms. It was like changing out the Bandaid without treating the wound below. Future doctors weren't trained to diagnose the root cause of underlying conditions that led to disease. Horrified, I wasn't willing to accept it. *I had to deactivate the ticking time bomb before it exploded, taking my father down with it.*

I researched, visited experts, and made calls to clinics all over the globe. I was making headway when, three weeks in, I developed debilitating headaches, panic attacks, social anxiety, depression, and digestive issues with a splash of hypochondria. My body was out of whack! Just about ready to test drive anything to ease my suffering, ironically, I became my very own guinea pig. As my father got better, my mother pleaded with me, "Please go see Dr. Soandso!" Reluctantly and out of respect, I went only to appease her. After the routine intake, he offered me the same prescriptions my father turned down, minus the pain meds. I left that appointment, simultaneously letting go of my fear, skepticism, and self-doubt.

Trusting my instincts, I opened up to the ancient wisdom of plant medicine to guide my health journey. Herbs not only brought my body back to balance, but they freed me from getting stuck in the pill for every ill model of today's healthcare system. I'm forever grateful for that difficult time. Without it, I don't know where I'd be. Sometimes, illness poses a meaningful lesson more valuable than finding the cure. My father lived well for over a decade past the doctor's prediction. Some say it was a miracle; I say it was his faith in nature, perseverance, and patience. His resilience inspired me to keep striving and spread knowledge to the rest of the world. Mother Nature taught me invaluable health skills I use within my family and share with my clients. I married a brilliant and loving pharmacist who aligned with me and embraced caring for our beloved patients through education and support. Together, we opened Vitahealth Apothecaries in New York City, where we continue to advise our community on how to best reach their optimal health goals.

THE SKILL

UTILIZING PLANT MEDICINE

Our bodies consist of trillions of cells, many of which we regenerate. We're constantly repairing and renewing ourselves. A medical professional has spent countless hours studying the human body and dividing it into all its parts. Many doctors believe a disease stems from one of those parts that needs to be dealt with apart from the rest. I believe we are the sum of our parts, mind, body, and soul, working in unison to produce the harmonious individual creations we call self.

Plant medicine has been used throughout different cultures for hundreds of thousands of years. It's nothing new, but we often need reminders. Herbs contain a myriad of biologically active constituents like alkaloids, flavonoids, phenolic acids, terpenes, tannins, and essential oils. These phytochemicals may treat various health conditions while supporting overall wellness. Herbs are available in different forms. There are edible herbs you can grow right in your home or purchase at the supermarket, like peppermint, basil, parsley, dill, cilantro, and rosemary. These are therapeutic, dried, or fresh. There are also more concentrated forms of herbs, such as those contained within certain supplement formulas, tinctures, extracts, oils, and powders.

Herbs are also commonly used in topical skincare products, as well as essential oils typically used for aromatherapy. Whichever way you welcome them into your life, having access to an herbal pharmacy at your fingertips empowers you to become a proactive part of your own health journey. Botanical medicine is multifaceted, science-backed, and effective. It's as versatile as it is powerful by enhancing the flavor of your recipes while replenishing vitality and restoring whole-body wellness. Using herbs in the kitchen is a great way to incorporate botanical medicine into your daily life. It's a valuable investment for the entire family. Herbs should be stored in dark, air-tight containers away from heat to maintain their freshness and potency. We keep a dedicated herbal cupboard at home with rows of labeled amber-colored glass mason jars.

Get your kids involved by bringing them along to food shop. Allow them to add personalized touches to their meals. It can be as easy as sprinkling some cinnamon on French toast. They find it pretty cool to rip off a few mint leaves to add to their tea or drinking water. It makes kids feel good to be included and gives them authority over what they put into their bodies. This practice encourages awareness and sets a healthy foundation that will follow them into adulthood. A quick disclaimer: I'm not a medical doctor; the information I'm sharing stems from years of research and personal experiences. It's for your educational purposes. With that in mind, drink and source your herbs responsibly! Purchase from reputable distributors to avoid consuming adulterated products, which can lead to undesirable side effects. Try to make sure your herbs are grown in clean, mineral-rich soil. Also, please err on the side of caution if you're pregnant, nursing, or taking prescription medications.

STRESS-REDUCING HERBS:

Stress leads to real physiological issues; let's be real, who's not stressed out? Plant medicines nourish, tone, soothe, and help your body adapt to daily stressors. The following herbs are referred to as nervines. Unlike traditional medications, which can lead to dependence and unwanted side effects, nervines strengthen connections between the nerves to restore healthy nervous system functioning. Excellent at alleviating anxiety while promoting relaxation, they're commonly used in combinations for synergistic effects. You can make tea infusions at home using fresh or dried herbs steeped in boiling water for 20-30 minutes. If you need something more immediately, take the tinctures or capsules. Some common spices like saffron and coriander are rich in antioxidants, B vitamins, and magnesium, an electrolyte essential for healthy nerves. These spices can also be added to boiling water to make a calming tea in a pinch.

1. **Passionflower (Passiflora incarnata)** is calming, sedating, and great for people who can't fall asleep due to an overactive mind. It also works for tension headaches, neuralgia, and anxiety.

2. **Lemon Balm (Melissa officinalis)** can quickly shift someone out of a stressed and depressed state, bad mood, irritability, and agitation. It's also useful in people who are prone to waking through the night. A wonderfully soothing herb for kids in the evenings given as a tea or alcohol-free tincture without being overly sedating.

3. **Chamomile (Matricaria recutita)** comes in many therapeutic varieties, such as English, Hungarian, German, and Roman. Chamomile is gentle yet highly effective for relieving anxiety and inducing relaxation. Rich in antioxidants, it activates the immune system and works well as an anti-infective, anti-spasmodic, and anti-inflammatory. It's commonly used to calm down teething pain in babies when rubbed on their gums. You can also freeze chamomile to make ice pops; This can come in handy for younger children. People with ragweed allergies should steer clear.

4. **Skullcap (Scutellaria laterfolia)** reduces ticks and tremors, improves circulation, aids sleep, and calms the nervous system. Skullcap is particularly helpful for people who are high-strung, hyperactive, or easily agitated.

5. **Valerian (Valeriana officinalis)** induces sedation, making it a useful aid for insomnia, nervousness, muscle spasms, cramping, PMS, and general stress. It's also indicated for irregular and rapid heartbeat.

IMMUNE BUILDING HERBS:

Many of nature's botanicals help stimulate a healthy immune response and promote overall health. The following herbs are especially beneficial during cold and flu season. They make amazing home cold remedies!

1. **Andrographis (Andrographis paniculata)** is a strong anti-viral, anti-parasitic, and anti-bacterial herb. A potent immune restorative, it reduces the severity and duration of sore throat, the common cold, and influenza. It's also cardioprotective, hepatoprotective and supports lung health.

2. **Garlic** is a natural disease fighter with multiple uses in the kitchen and the human body. Active compounds in garlic are called allicins. They're antibacterial, antiviral, anti-fungal, anti-parasitic, and treat a whole host of conditions. The advantages of eating garlic are everything from enhancing the immune system to shortening the duration of the common cold by half to preventing heart disease and lowering the risk of developing colorectal cancer.

3. **Oregano** is rich in powerful antioxidants. This culinary herb has high antimicrobial activity against viral, bacterial, and fungal infections. It also protects the body against food-borne pathogens like E. coli, Salmonella, and Listeria. To help combat a cold, I prefer taking oregano oil-filled capsules three times a day until symptoms subside. In the kitchen, I let my kids use it liberally in their soups, salads, and chicken dishes.

4. **Rosehips**, the berry part of the rose flower, is one of the richest forms of vitamin C known in nature. For those with healthy kidneys, Rosehips are fantastic taken throughout the winter months to help stave off viruses and keep the immune system robust. A handful of dried berries steeped in hot water makes a delicious tea.

5. **Mullein (Verbascum thapsus)** is rich in soothing mucin and immune-boosting saponins, which work together to exhibit an expectorant effect by coating the protective lining of the epithelium

in your respiratory tract. Mullein is often used to alleviate cough, bronchitis, and post-nasal drip caused by infections or irritants in the environment. Mullein flowers, combined with crushed garlic in a base of tea tree and olive oils, soothes earaches and treats Otitis Media.

DIGESTIVE HERBS:

Anyone with kids knows what it's like to hear "My tummy hurts" at 9 pm. Having some easy-to-use herbal remedies at home will make these troubles less taxing. Herbs that are safe, effective, and have a long history of use as medicine treating digestive upset include *Chamomile, Peppermint, Slippery elm,* and the roots of *Ginger, Marshmallow, Licorice,* and *Dandelion.* They promote healing of the gut lining and assist with Gastro Esophageal Reflux Disease (GERD), Dyspepsia, Irritable Bowel Syndrome (IBS), colitis, ulcers, spasms, diarrhea, constipation, bloating, and gastritis.

You might not realize that some medicinal plants are already in your refrigerator or on your spice rack. Since gut health begins in the mouth, it's nice to know herbs like *basil, parsley, cilantro, mint, ginger, rosemary,* and *fennel* have carminative, detoxifying, anti-spasmodic, and digestive benefits. I love adding fresh fennel to salads or using the seeds in cooking to make heavier meals more digestible. Fennel seeds can be chewed, crushed, or ground down into a powder.

1. **Marshmallow root (Althea officinalis)** is rich in thick, sticky mucilage that coats the intestinal tract to help reduce irritation and soothe symptoms of gastric upset. You can use loose herbs to make tea at home or bring encapsulated herbs along when on the go.

2. **Licorice root (Glycyrrhiza glabra)** is an excellent demulcent that soothes the mucosal lining of the lungs, bladder, stomach, and intestines. It's useful for heartburn, irritable bowel syndrome, and healing of stomach ulcers. It's best when used in combination with other herbs. In supplement form, it's known as DGL (deglycyrrhizinated licorice), which does not negatively impact blood pressure and is better for hypertensive people than regular licorice root herb.

3. **Peppermint (Mentha piperita)** leaves are spasmolytic because they work directly on the smooth muscle of the digestive tract to help ease cramps and spasms. Peppermint is a great carminative with antimicrobial effects. Peppermint oil capsules are commonly prescribed as an analgesic to relieve headaches and symptoms of IBS or indigestion. Studies have shown efficacy in IBS, upper respiratory tract, and gastrointestinal tract inflammation with symptoms including cramping, flatulence, gastritis, enteritis, nausea, and dyspepsia.

4. **Slippery elm (Ulmas rubra)** derives its name from the mucilaginous inner bark of the North American Elm tree. It's used for a vast array of complaints, from indigestion to bronchitis. Slippery elm is a highly nutritious herb effective at healing various tissues in the body. Its anti-inflammatory and soothing properties aid in coating the lining of the stomach, esophagus, intestinal wall, and lungs. The fiber-rich mucilage helps rid the body of unwanted toxins and may, in that way, work as a mild laxative. I always keep a packet of slippery elm lozenges in my bag. They're great for any stomach upset and come strawberry flavored, which my kids love!

5. **Dandelion root (Taraxacum officinale)** is a powerful bitter tonic rich in prebiotics that stimulate healthy gut flora, boost digestion, and relieve constipation. It's also commonly prescribed to improve liver function, reduce water retention, balance hormones, and regulate blood sugar levels.

REMEDY RECIPES:

Sore throat tea: 8 oz of hot water + 1-inch piece peeled and sliced ginger + 1/4 teaspoon powdered licorice root + 1 teaspoon powdered marshmallow root + 1 teaspoon Manuka honey + juice of 1 lemon + dash of cinnamon. Mix well before drinking.

Flu bomb tea: 8 oz of hot water + 1-2 cloves crushed garlic + 1/4 teaspoon ginger + 1/4 teaspoon cayenne pepper + 1/4 teaspoon grated turmeric root + juice of 1 whole lemon +1 teaspoon Manuka honey

Colic-ease infusion: 8 oz hot water + 1-inch piece peeled ginger + 1 teaspoon chamomile + 8 fresh dill branches + 1 handful fresh mint or 1

teaspoon dried herb + 1/4 teaspoon fennel seeds. For younger children, add a sprinkle of cinnamon and a bit of honey to lessen the bitterness. Steep for 15 minutes, strain, and sip slowly. A condensed version of this recipe may also be prepared by boiling fresh dill and fennel for 5-7 minutes, strain, and drink the herb water once cooled down. It's safe and effective for adults and kids of all ages.

Instant Relief Tummy tea: 8 oz hot water + 1 tablespoon of powdered Slippery elm + 1 teaspoon of powdered Marshmallow root. Stir thoroughly and drink while it's warm.

Slippery elm Porridge: For a vitamin-packed breakfast, mix one tablespoon of powdered slippery elm with one cup of warm nut milk and mix well until you get a slurry. Add in a handful of blueberries, a dash of cinnamon, 1/4 teaspoon of vanilla extract, and maple syrup. Healthy crunchy toppings can be gluten-free granola or some crushed nuts.

Pro tip: Capsaicin, the active ingredient in cayenne pepper, can quickly dilate and relax blood vessels, improving circulation. It also works like a styptic, stopping bleeding both internally and externally. Keep this powdered spice in your kitchen in case of cuts or emergencies.

When making herbal teas at home, be mindful to keep liquid intake to a minimum after 5 PM so your bladder doesn't interrupt your sleep.

I hope you enjoyed a small chapter of my life. Learn to listen to your body before the alarm goes off. You're a product of your environment, and lucky for you, herbal healers surround you. Get outdoors, feel the sun, inhale deeply, walk barefoot on grass, keep good company, be mindful, practice moderation, never stop learning, and love yourself unconditionally. Life is precious, have faith, show gratitude, stay humble, and have trust in your journey. I wish you all an abundance of health.

With my deepest gratitude and greatest pleasure,

Elina

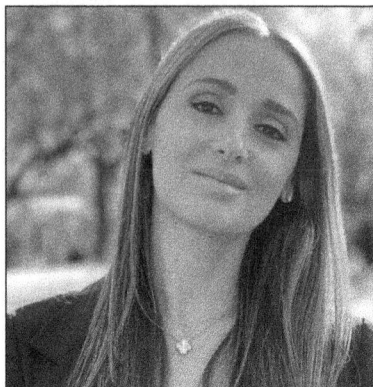

Elina K. Restrepo, RPh, ND, CNC, is a dedicated Pharmacist with over two decades of pharmaceutical and integrative health industry experience. She is a certified nutritional consultant, herbalist, and Naturopathic doctor. Elina is the CEO of Vitahealth Apothecaries in New York City. Together with her husband, David, they focus on patient-centric care via individualized regimens for fully holistic solutions to complex issues. Elina implements traditional medicines with non-traditional evidence-based nutritional supplements in her approach to treating various health concerns for the best possible outcomes. She leads the research and development sector of supplement formulations for private nutraceutical companies. Elina works collaboratively with functional medicine practitioners, applying various modalities for a number of health conditions. Over the years, she has contributed to several publications, including Weill Cornell Medical College Women's Health Advisor, Healthy Foods; Facts Vs. Fiction. She co-authored 21; 2 Experts 1 Goal, a book on healthy weight management. Elina currently serves as chief pharmacist representing IntraBio, a biopharmaceutical company developing medicines for rare genetic pediatric disorders and neurodegenerative diseases. She is a blessed mom of two remarkable children, who she describes as the main motivators that give her true purpose in her life. Elina resides in New York City with her three favorite humans and their clingy Cavapoo, Rocky. Her motto is "It's okay to be perfectly imperfect." In her free time, Elina enjoys early morning walks in the city, hot matcha lattes, pilates, traveling, and snuggling up with her kids on movie nights.

Connect with Elina:

Website: https://www.vitahealthapothecary.com

Email: elina@vitahealthapothecary.com

Instagram: https://www.Instagram.com/vitahealthapothecary

CHAPTER 12

SKIN

YOUR FIRST LINE OF DEFENSE

Eyal Levit, MD, FAAD, FACMS

MY STORY

I never imagined my journey to becoming a healer would begin in a small lab with bubbling colorful test tubes, Petri dishes filled with human skin cells, a radiation tag on my clothes, and an aroma of putrid chemicals that stung the eyes unless examined behind a protective shield inside a large and noisy ventilated hood at Columbia Presbyterian Hospital in Harlem. In that lab, during my college summer vacations, while testing the effects of pollutants and ultraviolet radiation on the skin, I found my calling under the mentorship of one of the world's leading researchers in photosensitivity disorders and allergic skin reactions, Dr. Vincent DeLeo.

The work fascinated me. I was surrounded by case studies of people who developed unexpected allergies to everyday chemicals found in everything from topical skin care products such as shampoos and moisturizers to implantable devices. I watched as the identification of these allergens transformed the lives of patients. Still, one question gnawed at me: Why do only some people get the reaction suddenly, often years after exposure to the allergen without any problem, and could we prevent these reactions from happening in the first place?

This curiosity led me down a path beyond just treating skin disorders— it pushed me toward a quest for prevention. I didn't want to be merely reactive; I wanted to be proactive in teaching people how to defend their skin from unhealthy environmental exposures while benefiting from healthy ones. My mission as a healer became clear: I needed to educate others about the importance of maintaining the health of their skin—our body's largest organ— and training it to become more resilient and healthier over time instead of broken and diseased.

To unwind at home after long hours in the lab, I read old classics, one of which was Homer's *Odyssey*. As I read about the weary and shipwrecked Odysseus being anointed with oil to help him revive, I wondered if this ancient practice had a scientific basis. Could we use certain natural oils to heal and protect the skin? I recalled my grandfather's daily ritual of massage and moisturizers and his almost legendary youthful vigor despite his age and arduous life. Little did I know, these ancient texts, coupled with my life experience, would lead me down a scientific discovery that would culminate in developing a system to help my patients' skin become a bastian of health and vigor that could withstand many of the pollutants I was battling in the lab while remaining flawless.

THE SKILL

THE SCIENCE—UNDERSTANDING YOUR AMAZING SKIN AND ITS ENVIRONMENT

Your skin is your body's largest organ, like a superhero shield protecting you from the outside world! It keeps germs out, helps you stay cool (maintaining the best temperature for your body's function), and even lets you feel things. Like a thermostat checking the outside weather, it constantly communicates with your command center in the brain to maintain a healthy body temperature. A highly sensitive alarm system wires the entire perimeter of the skin's border, activating your immune system when the perimeter is compromised or intruders try to break in. The inside of our cells is made of 80% water. To function properly, this concentration must be maintained. Any damage to the cell wall from chemicals, sun, smoke, or physical forces may result in over-drying, overheating, or physical breakdown, leading to the loss of that water, death of the cells, and activation of the skin's alarm system and its immunity.

YOUR SKIN IS MADE OF LAYERS LIKE A CAKE

Your skin has three main layers: the top layer (epidermis), a middle layer (dermis), and a bottom layer (underneath the dermis made of fat and muscle called subqutis), all layered over and glued to your bones that house and protect your vital organs. Think of it like a delicious layer cake but for your body—a delicious and beautiful cake covered with hard, detailed decorations on its top. The hair and nails give your skin a unique flavor and are made of a harder protein, unlike the soft one that makes up your skin.

YOUR MICROBIOME

Your body does not exist in a vacuum. Over millions of years, it has cultivated friendly relationships with good bacteria, offering them a nutritious, safe home. In return, the bacteria jealously guard their turf and, like a friendly army, keep bad bacteria, fungi, and viruses away. This friendly army promises to defend the skin and not attack the layers under the skin as long as the skin keeps its part of the bargain and maintains the integrity of the friendly upper layer (epidermis) that comprises their home, their microbiome. These tiny helpers are like an invisible secret defense layer covering your skin, airways, and gut. When you wash your skin too much or use harsh soaps, you can hurt this friendly army, making your skin dry, itchy, and prone to bad bacteria and infections.

GLANDULAR AND IMMUNE HEALTH

The middle layer of the skin contains many of the small piping systems supplying the upper layer of the skin and its invisible defending army. These pipes are called glands—eccrine, apocrine, and sebaceous—which exit through the upper layer of the skin and contribute to the body's cooling system, odor, and skin lubrication, respectively. Sometimes, these pipes get clogged, leading to pimples. Proper hygiene and maintenance of these glands prevent the overgrowth of unhealthy bacteria, which, if unchecked, can penetrate deeper and lead to infections or allergic reactions. Other pipes supply nutrition and remove waste products; they are called arteries, veins, and lymphatic vessels.

THE SKIN'S POLICE SYSTEM

Although the skin has a friendly army of bacteria on its outside borders, it maintains a standing police force that constantly patrols its undersurface. This police force is part of our army, called the immune system. The immune system also plays a role in skin health. If the healthy balance of bacteria on our skin surface is disrupted, or an intruder is recognized breaking through the upper skin layer, the immune system is affected, and a war ensues; medically, this war is called inflammation. Conditions like cradle cap (a yellow-golden, flaky, thick crust on the baby's head), caused by the overgrowth of yeast on the scalp, presenting as dandruff in later adulthood, are examples of how the immune system reacts to changes in its external microbiome. Proper shampooing to keep this yeast away is a simple remedy that is sadly often overlooked.

BALANCING THE OUTSIDE ENVIRONMENT: THE SUN—HEALER OR KILLER?

To understand how to care for the skin, we must first recognize that the environment influences its health. UV (ultraviolet) light exposure, pollution, and harsh chemicals can disrupt its natural balance. The sun is powerful, like a super-bright light! A little light is needed to see, but if there is too much bright light, you are blinded. Like our sight, our skin layers and their structures are similarly affected by the sun. Too much sun, and our skin is damaged, and our circulating police forces (immune cells) are lulled to sleep (suppressed) by its radiation; too little, and we lose its benefits such as warmth, disinfection, and the production of our happy messengers (hormones like serotonin and dopamine) and vitamins like Vitamin D.

Damage to skin cells from the sun or other environmental pollutants forces the body to produce new cells to replace them in the skin's outer wall of defense. Eventually, the body becomes exhausted and fails to produce good-quality, functioning skin cells, and damaged cells that can become cancerous may form. That's why it's so important to maintain and protect your skin—your first line of defense.

PRACTICAL PEARLS

Help Me Help You.

Here are simple steps to avoid a common problem my patients experience—dry, itchy, bleeding, painful skin. We often think that drinking water is enough to hydrate the skin, but our skin loses moisture to the environment. This is why environmental control and external hydration through skincare is just as crucial as internal hydration.

The Importance of Skin Microbiome and Hydration

Maintaining the balance of the skin microbiome—a community of microorganisms living on the skin—is vital for its overall health. Disruptions to this balance, through harsh skincare routines or over-washing, can weaken the skin's barrier, leading to dryness, irritation, and increased susceptibility to infections or allergic reactions. To combat this, one must cleanse gently, hydrate properly, and maintain a healthy surrounding environment.

1. **Be Cool:** *Wash With Cool Water* When waking up, use cool water without soap or cleansers to wash your face and neck in the sink. I also like to wet my shoulders and arms and spread some cool water on the rest of my body. Cool water helps keep your healthy oils while activating your epidermis (upper skin layer) thermostat system to signal the brain about the outside environment. This cool signal causes the body to produce energy to warm the skin, giving the skin a needed boost of energy to stay young and healthy.

Shower daily with short showers and cool water. Always opt for cool water over hot. Hot water strips away the skin's natural oils and can compromise its barrier, making it more vulnerable to irritants and allergens that can activate its police system, leading to inflammation. Showers should be kept to five minutes to prevent degreasing of the skin. For babies, five minutes in a basin or bath is also sufficient to keep their skin healthy without disrupting the natural oils.

2. **Clean and Heal—Strip, and You'll Trip:** The art of proper, gentle skin cleansing. Using your hands, instead of a washcloth or a sponge, wash your body with cool water using gentle, fragrance-free soaps only in key areas where bacteria accumulate, such as the armpits, groin, and folds of the skin. The rest of your skin can be washed

effectively with water alone. This keeps the upper skin layer and the immune system healthy, prevents striping your healthy cells, and maintains a clean, healthy skin barrier, glandular piping system, and continuous supply of natural oils that protect the skin barrier and the friendly bacteria defending it.

3. **Schmear It to Clear It—Hydration After Cleansing:** After a shower, one should gently "squeegee" off excess water with their hands, much like wiping a windshield. Immediately afterward, while the skin is still wet, apply a hydrating oil, such as a Tuscan massage oil. Since water and oil do not mix, applying the oil over your wet skin locks in moisture, keeping the skin supple and giving additional protection not only to the skin but also to the friendly bacteria defending it. The act of massaging the oil into the skin not only hydrates but also stimulates blood flow, benefiting all the layers of your tasty cake from the upper two layers of the skin with its pipes to its third layer comprised of the fat, muscles and nerves coursing through it. The process doesn't need to end there—air drying or using a blow dryer can remove any residual oiliness without losing moisture. This routine also applies to the scalp, where massage oil can be applied the night before, especially for babies. This helps heal the scalp and protect it from irritants and pollutants. In the morning, the oil can be gently washed off, promoting a healthy scalp without causing acne. Based on my personal experience and clinical practice, using massage oil on the scalp has not led to acne or skin occlusion, even in those prone to breakouts.

4. **Practice Makes Perfect:** repeat the process ideally three times per day. Wet the skin with cool water, apply a moisturizing oil or ointment over the wet skin. If the skin is still dry add another layer of lubrication over the oil using a small amount of a thick moisturizer like *Aquaphor Original Ointment*, the less ingredients the better.

5. **Maintaining Humidity and Moisturizing Sensitive Areas:** Another key to skin health is maintaining a healthy environment. Indoor humidity should be set around 55% to prevent the air from becoming too dry, which can strip the skin of moisture, or too humid, which can encourage the growth of mold or fungus. Moisturizing the nostrils and ears with a small amount of oil or Aquaphor can prevent

dryness in these sensitive areas, especially in arid climates or during the winter months. Make sure to use clean hands and avoid pushing anything deeper than the nostril's opening.

ANCIENT WISDOM MEETS MODERN SCIENCE— COMING FULL CIRCLE

Skincare is not just a modern concern. The ancient Greeks and Romans knew about the benefits of oil on the skin. In Homer's *Odyssey*, Odysseus was washed ashore and anointed with oil, a practice kings underwent for centuries as recorded in the Bible to have been done by Moses to Aaron, his brother and other high priests (Exodus 30:26), and later to priests and kings in Israel over 1000 BCE. These age-old rituals of oil application weren't just about appearance—they were about protection, hydration, and healing. Our modern understanding aligns with this ancient wisdom: oils can seal in moisture, restore skin pH, and provide a barrier against environmental irritants. As we say at Levit Dermatology, Health and Beauty is Our Duty. Be Good, Do Good, and May Good Come Your Way.

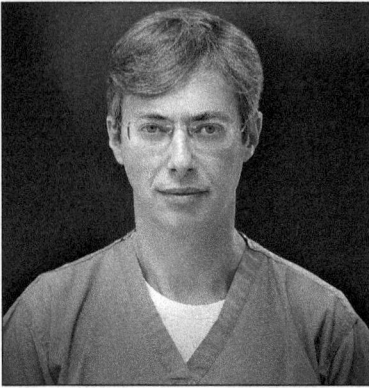

Dr. Eyal Levit is a board-certified dermatologist and cosmetic surgeon with over 27 years of experience. As the director of a cosmetic surgery fellowship and an associate professor at Columbia Presbyterian Hospital and Mount Sinai Hospitals, Dr. Levit has received many accolades, including the Best Teacher of the Year award by the Mount Sinai/St. Luke's Hospital dermatology residents and has dedicated his career to advancing skin health through preventive care and cutting-edge treatments. Known for his expertise in addressing photosensitivity, cosmetic, and skin cancer treatment, Dr. Levit continues to educate patients and colleagues alike on how to best protect the skin from environmental hazards. Dr. Levit holds patents in treating Type 1 Diabetes and designs in air purification devices developed during the Covid pandemic. He has authored both lay and medical textbooks and has presented around the world on innovations in dermatology and cosmetic surgery, contributing to global discussions on longevity, skincare, and wellness.

Dr. Levit is currently starring in a reality TV series called "Skin Deep with Dr. Levit: Beyond the Skin" airing on doctorTVNetwork available on Roku and other streaming platforms.

Connect with Dr. Levit:

Website: https://Levitdermatology.com

Instagram: https://www.instagram.com/levitdermatology and
https://www.instagram.com/levitcosmetics

Facebook: https://www.facebook.com/levitdermatology

Youtube: www.youtube.com/@levitdermatology1939

CHAPTER 13

TOXIC OVERWHELM

PRACTICAL STRATEGIES
TO REDUCE THE HARM

Emily Givler, DSC

MY STORY

It was 2018. I was building my practice as a Functional Genomic Nutrition Consultant. The non-profit I volunteered with had just done some exciting research on pesticide residue in food and breast milk that was getting a lot of attention. I lectured at conferences around the country. And at home I took all the steps I could to avoid environmental toxins because I was a crunchy mom of three.

My children, I told myself, *will grow up with the benefits of everything I know about the poisons in our food and water. I'll keep them safe.*

Safe from PFAS, the forever chemicals. Safe from plastics. Safe from perchlorate, phthalates, and pesticides. Safe from the sea of toxins making kids all around them sick with hormonal disruptions and developmental delays. With allergies. ADHD. Autism. Cancer. I did everything I could to dodge them all.

I read labels. I filtered our water. I knew my farmers by name. I made our meals from scratch. I eliminated my teflon pots and pans. I used natural products around the house and yard. I eliminated artificial fragrances. I felt a little overwhelmed and paranoid. *But at least my kids would be safe.*

Because I wasn't just a crunchy mom. It was part of my job to know the science, to read the papers, to give the lectures. I understood that phthalates can alter children's delicate developing endocrine systems, changing their hormones. I knew the profound neurotoxicity of organophosphate pesticides. I spent my days analyzing genetic variants that impacted the clearance of toxic compounds. *Are you paranoid if the things you're worried about are real?*

That year, while attending an environmental medicine conference, I decided to run some toxin testing on my kids. I didn't expect to find much but I thought it would be a good tool for evaluating all my crunchy efforts. I was thoroughly unprepared for the results.

"N-acetyl (3,4-dihydroxybutyl) cysteine." That was a mouthful. There were extremely high levels in my three-year-old and low levels in my school-aged children. I read the report details. "Evidence of exposure to synthetic rubber." "Primary route of exposure is through inhalation." "Some exposure may occur through dermal contact." "Known carcinogen."

I read those results, and I knew. It was the playground. His ***favorite*** playground. The one we went to when his big brother and sister were at school. The one with recycled rubber tire mulch that cushioned those little toddler falls. It seemed like such a good idea! A way to reduce trash in landfills, give the tires a second life on playgrounds and athletic fields across the country. All those bits of rubber baking in the sun, off-gassing into the atmosphere for all those little lungs to breathe in. And I missed it.

That test shook me. It highlighted how truly widespread these contaminants are. My children were healthy. I hadn't tested them because they were sick or having problems. I tested them because I'm a big, curious nerd with access to testing. I did what I thought were ***all the things*** to keep my kids safe from the sea of toxins they were swimming in, yet they were still being poisoned by the world around them. If my child, protected by all of my knowledge, could still have this extreme exposure, what about other kids whose parents didn't think about these things all the time? In my case, we could avoid this toxin. We could seek out playgrounds with wooden mulch instead of its rubber counterpart. But what if we hadn't run the test? And what if it wasn't that easy to get away from the toxin?

The reality is not everyone is this lucky. Sometimes, the toxins are in our homes. Sometimes, they're in our food, water, or air. Sometimes, they're incredibly persistent in our bodies. Not everyone stays healthy with this level of exposure. I know firsthand from my work that some individuals are more vulnerable to bioaccumulation of specific toxins than others, often because of genetic vulnerabilities along critical detox pathways. I see every day what happens when an environmental toxic exposure runs up against a weak pathway: a greater potential for negative health impacts. These individuals can be thought of as canaries in our collective coal mine, highlighting the extreme dangers of these toxins at lower levels than might affect the general population.

Our bodies have an intricate network of organs and systems that work together to detoxify the compounds we encounter day to day. The liver works in two phases to bio-transform fat-soluble toxins into a water-soluble form that can be eliminated in sweat, urine, or stool. Beyond just the liver, the kidneys and lymphatics work together to filter toxins and impurities. People with genetic weakness along any portion of these pathways may be more vulnerable to a buildup of specific toxins and their negative health effects. Before we were exposed to thousands of synthetic chemicals, those systems, even the genetically vulnerable ones, could largely keep up with the toxic input. Now, our daily exposure is so great we're starting to see health impacts regardless of our genes.

It's important to note that there are dozens of biochemical pathways that play a role in biotransformation and detoxification. The skills discussed here can be helpful broadly, but if you're struggling with significant exposure or challenges trying to detox, working with a knowledgeable practitioner may allow you to take a more targeted and nuanced approach.

THE SKILL

IDENTIFYING AND REDUCING THE TOXIC LOAD

We can't change something if we don't know it needs changing. Understanding that many of our chemical exposures are tied to many contemporary health challenges, like rising rates of allergies, ADHD, and pediatric cancers, is the first step. From here, we need to empower ourselves with the knowledge of not only what's out there but what we can do about it.

There is an ever-growing body of evidence showing that the toxins in our environment have a negative impact on human health. This isn't a new idea. In 1962, Rachel Carson published *Silent Spring*, introducing the idea that poisons in our environment do not remain in their intended targets; they travel through food chains. We've been shown time and time again in the decades since that we're part of those food chains. We're part of our ecosystem. What we pour into our environment, we ultimately take back up into ourselves. This knowledge hasn't stopped us from developing over 350,000 man-made chemicals, seeking "better living through chemistry." It makes life so cheap and convenient! Nonstick cookware. Single-serve packaging. Waterproof clothing. Life could be so easy! We've now had decades of ever-increasing chemical exposures, and we're living with the long-term cost of that short-term convenience. It turns out there's nothing easy about developmental delays and behavioral problems. There's nothing cheap about cancer.

It's shocking to discover how new and widespread this problem is. Our children face a far greater chemical burden than previous generations. Half of all plastic on the planet has been produced since 2005. Worldwide agricultural use of pesticides continues to increase, reaching 3.69 million metric tons annually as of 2022. Globally, chemical production has increased 50-fold since the 1950s, much of that due to the proliferation of PFAS, often referred to as "forever chemicals" because of their environmental persistence. The toxic burden continues to grow. We can't stick our heads in the sand when it comes to this reality. We've pushed the limits of what we can handle, and the cost is the health of future generations.

Are you feeling overwhelmed yet?

When it comes to building awareness of the toxins impacting our health, it can quickly start to feel this way. Keep breathing. Focus on action steps. We're opening our eyes to this so that we can decrease exposure to increase our health. But where to start? A good strategy is to avoid the 3P's: Pesticides, Plastics, and PFAS. These three offenders are widespread and produce cumulative harm as exposure continues. Let's dig a little deeper into each.

PESTICIDES

Organophosphate pesticides can have significant adverse effects on the health of developing bodies, brains, and nervous systems. Chronic diseases linked to pesticide exposure range from various types of cancers to neurological disorders, developmental delays, and infertility. We're exposed to them in our food, water, and our air. When thinking about food, organic food is generally far lower in pesticide residue than its conventional counterpart. Transitioning to organics is a huge step in reducing pesticide exposure. The Environmental Working Group (EWG) publishes an annual Clean 15/ Dirty Dozen shopping guide at https://www.ewg.org/foodnews/dirty-dozen.php. It's a handy reference to keep track of which produce items are most heavily pesticide-treated, meaning most important to purchase organically when possible. It also lists the items that are safest to purchase conventionally so you can make informed choices while shopping to stretch your budget. In terms of water, filtration with certain activated charcoal filters and Reverse Osmosis (RO) treatment can reduce up to 100% of these contaminants. More on that later.

Beyond our water and food, pesticide exposure can happen at parks, playgrounds, athletic fields, and your own backyard. Those verdant spaces don't stay green on their own. A cocktail of chemicals is applied regularly to keep those fields weed-free. States have differing rules regarding pesticide application notifications. Most commonly, signs will be posted in the area where pesticide spraying is taking place to alert visitors. If there are areas you frequent, take the time to find out how they post their notifications and pay attention. Avoiding those spaces for 24-48 hours after application can greatly reduce exposure.

PLASTIC

This may prove to be one of the biggest sources of toxins for younger generations. Every bit of plastic ever produced is still here, broken down into progressively smaller pieces, dubbed micro and nano plastics. The small size of these plastic particulates makes them easy to transport in air and water cycles, meaning that regardless of where they originated, they've become a global problem. We find microplastics on every corner of the globe and, more concerningly, in every human tissue we study. It's in our lungs. It's in our brains. It's in semen. It's in the placentas of pregnant women. It's everywhere. Current estimates are that Americans ingest, on average, five grams of microplastics every week. That's a credit card's worth of plastic. Weekly. And we're beginning to learn that these plastics don't just sit harmlessly in our systems.

Most of us already know not to heat things in plastic. Solid advice. When heated, plastic toxins transfer into the surrounding food or liquid. We happen to be a nice toasty 98.6 degrees, which means those microplastics don't just hang out in our tissues. A growing number of studies show that the chemical components of plastics—namely phthalates and bisphenols—migrate from microplastics into us. In developing bodies, this can be particularly harmful. These chemicals are what are known as endocrine system disruptors. In plain language, they can majorly mess up hormones and hormone receptors in a variety of ways, ranging from fertility challenges to early puberty to increased risk of multiple forms of cancer. They're also associated with additional health problems, including increased risk of asthma, allergies, developmental and learning delays, and attention and behavioral difficulties in children.

One of the best strategies we can employ to reduce our exposure to microplastics is proper water filtration. Widespread testing has revealed that tap and bottled water both contain extremely high levels of microplastics. The good news is that charcoal filters and RO filtration can reduce the vast majority of microplastics in your home water, regardless of which brand you choose. Just be sure to filter your water into glass, not back into more plastic!

Minimizing single-use plastics, particularly in food packaging, is a way to reduce not only your family's exposure to phthalates and bisphenols but also a way to keep the global plastic burden from growing. As it stands, we're on track to double the amount of plastic on the planet again by 2040. Phasing out single-use plastics is important, but speaking from personal experience, make this a long-term strategy. Once you start paying attention to the plastic around you, you'll quickly realize just how ubiquitous it is. Accept that this is going to be a long-term project right from the get-go. Using resources like the Zero Waste Store can help streamline that process.

When it comes to diet, there is some evidence that eating a high amount of fiber, particularly in the form of resistant starch like plantains or cooked and cooled rice, may reduce the intake of microplastics from food. If you use sea salt at home, changing your salt source can also reduce your plastic intake, as most sea salt now contains microplastics. There are individual foods that have higher microplastic contamination than salt, but because of how much salt we use relative to other foods, changing it up can have a high impact. You can find some of my favorite resistant starch and clean salt sources on the book resource page.

PFAS

Per- and polyfluoroalkyl substances (PFAS) are a group of thousands of synthetic chemicals used in industrial and consumer products worldwide since the 1940s. Dubbed "forever chemicals," they're extremely persistent in the environment and in the human body, taking thousands of years to break down. They're found in nonstick cookware, water-repellent clothing, stain-resistant fabrics and carpets, lotions and cosmetics, firefighting foams, and products that resist grease, water, and oil. They're found in dental floss, disposable contacts, and 99% of bottled water. Their widespread use and their presence as a persistent contaminant in groundwater results in most people, about 97% in the United States, having been exposed.

These compounds are "presumed to be immune hazards to humans based on a high level of evidence," per the US National Toxicology Program. There is epidemiological evidence suggesting a link between exposure to certain PFAS and kidney and testicular cancers, liver damage, and pregnancy complications from pregnancy-induced hypertension and preeclampsia to decreased birth weight. And they are forever. Once they are in, we don't have good strategies to get them back out. There is some evidence that soluble fibers like psyllium husk and pectin may be beneficial, but our best strategy is avoidance. Water filtration is an important step in reducing exposure.

In addition to filtering your water, safe cookware is key for PFAS reduction. Nonstick cookware is a big source of home exposure. Use stainless steel, cast iron, or glass cookware instead. You should also be cautious with food packaging, especially take-out food containers. PFAS are commonly used here because of their water and grease resistance. This includes microwave popcorn bags, fast-food wrappers, and pizza boxes. Just like with plastic toxins, these poisons can migrate into your food. Using a resource like the free Detox Me app from the Silent Spring Institute can be a valuable tool as you work on phasing these chemicals out of your household. Find it here: https://silentspring.org/detox-me-app-tips-healthier-living.

In the bathroom, phase out PFAS exposure by avoiding personal care products with ingredients labeled "fluoro" or "perfluoro. These are often found in cosmetics like waterproof mascara and body lotion. Get help finding safer replacements here: https://pfascentral.org/pfas-free-products/.

PRIORITIZE

Are you feeling overwhelmed now? That's a mountain of toxins in all sorts of places and we've talked about a lot of changes you can make. Instead of trying to tackle everything at once, prioritize this high-impact change to minimize plastics, pesticides, and PFAS in one step.

The single most impactful strategy we can use to avoid all 3P's is proper water filtration. This one action carries a massively oversized benefit when it comes to reducing exposure to not only these harmful compounds but to a multitude of other pollutants that can be found in the majority of water sources. The right filter can reduce microplastics, PFAS, pesticides, heavy metals, and other pollutants. And no, your refrigerator filter doesn't cut it. So how do you know what to use?

My answer to the question of "What filter is best?" is always, "It depends on what's in your water." A practical solution for anyone in the United States who uses municipal water is the Environmental Working Group's Tap Water Database, found at https://www.ewg.org/tapwater/. This free database allows you to search by zip code to learn which contaminants are in your drinking water. Importantly, it also tells you what type of filter (carbon, reverse osmosis, or ion exchange) will most effectively reduce those specific toxins allowing you to make the right choice for your family.

In reality, for most municipal and well water, Reverse Osmosis is likely to be the optimal filtration option. If you're going this route, make sure you are re-mineralizing your water to restore the essential elements lost during the filtration process. Simply add a few drops of trace minerals into your water after filtering but before drinking. This is especially important for children's rapidly growing bones. It's much easier to put minerals back into filtered water than it is to get most of these toxins out of your body. You can find some of my favorite water filters and trace minerals on the Book Resource page at https://www.EmilyGivler.com

Once your water is properly filtered, work on implementing additional toxin-reduction strategies one step at a time. Focus next on what goes on and in your body like food and personal care products. Utilize the resources discussed to eliminate these poisons progressively. Remember: these toxins are cumulative and your efforts to eliminate them need to be as well.

PERFECTION

There's just one final "P" to avoid when it comes to reducing our toxic load: Perfection. Give up the idea of being perfect and focus on doing better. Accept that there will be things you miss. I completely missed the playground! Don't let those missteps stop you. You can do this. Your eyes are open now. Keep breathing. You *can* reduce the harm.

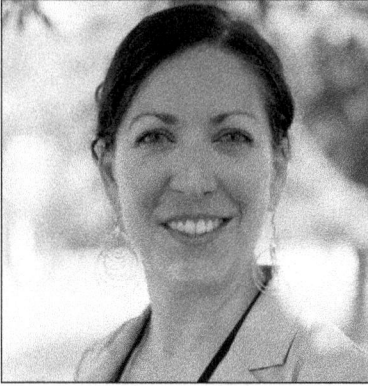

Emily Givler, DSC is a Functional/Genomic Nutrition Consultant, researcher, author, and lecturer with a thriving practice alongside her mentor, Bob Miller, at Tree of Life in Ephrata, Pennsylvania. She holds advanced certifications in Nutrition, Herbalism, and Nutrigenomic Analysis from the Holt Institute of Medicine, PanAmerican University of Natural Health, and the Nutrigenomic Research Institute, where she now serves as an advisor and supplement formulator. In her consulting practice, Emily develops personalized dietary and nutritional protocols based on genetic predispositions, environmental and epigenetic influences, and functional lab testing to help her clients optimize their health.

In addition to her clinical work, Emily is the co-founder of Beyond Protocols where she leads their mentorship team, teaching practitioners advanced integration of functional genomics into clinical practice. She also offers one-on-one practitioner mentoring, helping colleagues navigate the complex web of genetic polymorphisms to develop more effective protocols for their chronically ill or complex cases.

Emily's work as a researcher led to her collaboration with Drs. Neil Nathan and Beth O'Hara on Precision Mycotoxin Detoxification, which foundationally reshaped the way many practitioners approach mold detoxification. She continued her collaboration with Dr. Nathan as a contributing author in his 2024 book, The Sensitive Patient's Healing Guide: Top Experts Offer New Insights for Environmental Toxins, Lyme Disease, and EMFs.

In her personal life, Emily loves to hike, forage for medicinal and edible plants and fungi, and travel with her incredible children, who are the lights of her life.

Connect with Emily:

Websites:

www.TOLhealth.com

www.BeyondProtocols.org

www.EmilyGivler.com

YouTube:

https://www.youtube.com/@beyondprotocols5233

CHAPTER 14

POOP IS PIVOTAL

HOW ENERGY FLOW HELPS YOU GO

Heather Schuerlein, DACM, AP, FABORM, Dipl.OM

"If you don't take care of this most magnificent machine that you've ever been given, where are you going to live?"

~ Karyn Calabrese

MY STORY

"I can't live like this anymore." I'm used to hearing these words as an acupuncture physician and doctor of Chinese medicine. I've been in practice for almost 15 years now. When patients end up at my door they have usually exhausted all options. I like to say I'm the last resort with one of the best results.

I started this journey in holistic medicine when I was 27. I experienced an abnormally heavy, painful menstrual cycle. Each month, the pain was so bad I missed work and family events.

I felt like my life revolved around my menstrual cycle. Mainstream Western medicine didn't have any answers; just that, as a woman, it's what we have to "live with." The only option Western medicine gave me was birth control. I did try it for a month, but it also made me sick. Frustrated and tired of feeling like this, I went looking for answers. I didn't want to live like that anymore, but I had no idea what road to take. *How could I help myself feel better naturally?* I wondered.

Along my educational road, I met a woman who changed my life. Her name was Dr. MaryJoyce (MJ for short), and she was my anatomy and physiology teacher. She was also an extremely talented acupuncture and Chinese herbal medicine doctor.

"Acupuncture can help with many pain-related conditions," Dr. MJ mentioned in class one day. And in that moment I wondered—*can she help me?* I worked up the nerve to talk to her after class. I had a dirty secret that I didn't want anyone to know about. At that point in my life, I was a smoker, and I knew she'd be on my tush about it, being a health teacher.

She agreed to help me with my menstrual cycle, as well as help me quit smoking.

I saw her twice a week for acupuncture at her office. My acupuncture treatments were extremely calming, peaceful, and restful. Within one week, I noticed positive changes in my body: I slept better, pooped better, and I felt more calm. I stayed after class to chat with her about what I could expect to feel and how acupuncture and Chinese herbal medicine helped her other patients. I was fascinated.

During the first month of acupuncture treatments, I continued to sleep better, have amazing poops, have more energy, and most of all, my periods weren't nearly as painful. She gave me home exercises to do as well, certain foods to eat and what not to eat according to my constitution and Chinese medical diagnosis. I was instructed to use acupressure (the firm pressing of an acupuncture point) when I had pain at work.

"Press this point LI 4 firmly and hold for a minute. It will move your Qi and help with the pain," Dr. MJ instructed me. This piece of information saved me from missing work many times. It took a few months of consistent treatment, but eventually, the pain during my menstrual cycle was *gone*.

The reason I became a doctor of acupuncture and Chinese medicine was to help others the way Dr. MJ helped me.

I see a lot of patients with pain: neck pain, back pain, knee pain, and pain in the lower abdomen, usually due to constipation. One patient, let's call him Bob, came in for his acupuncture appointment because he hadn't had a bowel movement in a week. He looked a bit wary of the needles but was willing to try anything, especially something that could help him poop. Acupuncture was "woo woo" to him. After looking at his tongue and taking his pulse, I decided he needed a little bit of help in the movement department. I chose a very well-known point for the first needle, LI 4 (the hand point known for helping move things along). As Bob lay there, calm and relaxed (the room was filled with gentle music), he said, "I feel a warmth in my stomach." I nodded.

"Just rest now. I'll be back in 15 minutes to check on you," I told him.

At the 15-minute mark, I opened the door, and Bob's eyes shot wide open. "Uh, Doc, I think we need to speed this up," he whispered, clearly trying to maintain his composure.

As soon as the needles were fully removed, Bob raced to the restroom like an Olympic sprinter. I just chuckled, hearing Bob from the hallway joyously declaring, "I've been freed! It worked!"

Bob became a lifelong believer in acupuncture but now always double-checks how close the bathroom is before each session. Lucky for him, he always made it in time.

Just for the record, I've never had an "accident" in the office! Then there was George, a self-proclaimed skeptic of "all things woo-woo," who reluctantly agreed to try acupuncture for his constipation after his wife practically forced him into the clinic. He spent the first part of his consultation rolling his eyes and cracking jokes about "voodoo magic."

I patiently explained how acupuncture could help get things moving, and George sarcastically asked, "So, you stick me with a few needles, and I magically poop? Sure, doc, let's do it."

Thirty minutes later, after a session that included points like SJ 6 and LI 4, George got up, feeling surprisingly relaxed. He thanked me but still wasn't convinced. I smiled and said, "Give it a few hours."

Later that evening, George was at home watching TV when he suddenly bolted to the bathroom, where he stayed for quite a while. Emerging triumphantly, he emailed me: "You win, Doc. Magic needles: 1, George's constipation: 0." From that day forward, George became an acupuncture convert but would still jokingly refer to his sessions as "needle magic for the grumpy gut."

There are so many stories I can share, from husbands who were dragged into the office kicking and screaming to reluctant, skeptical people turning firm believers. There's nothing to believe in, though. Acupuncture, as old as it is, works through something even older: your nervous system.

UNDERSTANDING ACUPUNCTURE

In Chinese medicine, there are 14 (or 12, depending on who you talk to) major meridians in the body. In Chinese medicine, qi (pronounced "chee") is considered the vital life force or energy that flows through all living beings. It's believed to animate the body and maintain health and balance. Qi is what helps the digestive system break down food, helps blood flow through the circulatory system, and stimulates the bowels to release (with nice, healthy poops). Qi flows in specific pathways, known as meridians, which are like energetic highways that connect different parts of the body, including the organs, tissues, and systems.

When thinking about and trying to understand meridians, think of your nervous system. The central nervous system connects your brain to the rest of your body, the peripheral nervous system connects your limbs with your central system. The autonomic nervous system has two branches: the sympathetic and parasympathetic. When qi is flowing smoothly and freely, the body is in a state of balance, leading to good health and vitality.

Our qi flow gets clogged when we get out of balance. Think about how you feel when you go on vacation and eat and drink excessively. You may get really hot; you may experience bloating, gas, or even constipation. When we eat and drink foods that are super rich and heavy, we block our digestive qi mechanism and our "wheel" doesn't turn. When that happens over a long period of time, symptoms such as acid reflux, anxiety, foggy-headedness, and constipation can develop.

By stimulating specific points along the meridians, called acupoints, practitioners help the qi move more effectively through the body, promoting healing, pain relief, and improved overall well-being. Now that we know what meridians are and how they connect to each organ or organ system let's talk about how you can help constipation with acupuncture (or acupressure).

Acupuncture/acupressure is highly beneficial for chronic constipation because it addresses the root causes of the condition by restoring balance to the body's Qi (energy) and enhancing the function of the digestive system. In Chinese medicine, chronic constipation is seen as a result of imbalances such as qi stagnation, deficiency of qi, blood, or yin, or excessive heat in the digestive organs. To put this in plain words, constipation is either due to a deficiency, excess, or disharmony. It's not just the constipation; it's the *type* of constipation. Acupuncture helps by stimulating specific points along the body's meridians to regulate these imbalances and promote better digestion and elimination.

Chronic stress or emotional imbalances can disrupt the flow of qi, leading to tension in the digestive organs and contributing to constipation. Acupuncture is effective at calming the mind, relieving stress, and regulating emotional imbalances that can worsen chronic constipation. By helping to relax the body and mind, acupuncture addresses one of the underlying causes of constipation related to emotional tension.

Chronic constipation often results from weakness or deficiency in the spleen or stomach qi, which leads to poor digestion and weak intestinal motility. Acupuncture points that tonify or strengthen the spleen and stomach help improve the body's ability to digest food and move waste through the intestines. This can lead to more regular bowel movements and softer stools. When your spleen or stomach qi is weak, it's like your digestive system is running low on fuel. This means your body doesn't have enough energy to keep things moving through your intestines the way it should.

Acupuncture helps increase peristalsis, the wave-like muscle contractions of the intestines that move stool through the digestive tract. When peristalsis is weak, it can lead to constipation. Acupuncture can promote these contractions, helping the body more efficiently eliminate waste.

What you eat and drink will also affect how your bowels move. Are you drinking enough water? The current guidelines say half your body weight in ounces of water per day. That means if you're 200 pounds, you should be drinking 100 ounces of water every day. I know it sounds like a lot! Think of it this way: if you don't "float the boat," the boat doesn't float. In other words, your poop boat is stuck at the dock with no water around to safely carry it to its next destination: your toilet. Foods that can be eaten to help with chronic constipation are pears, sesame seeds (tahini), figs, dates, bananas, sweet potatoes, oatmeal, almonds, and spinach. All pack a great amount of fiber to help get that boat moving.

When patients come to the office for treatment, I address the root cause of the problem as well as the constipation. A patient's treatment plan will include herbs, acupuncture, food suggestions, and probiotics to help their digestive system run smoothly. The points below will help you if you feel like you're a little sluggish. Please see my resource webpage for tips, tricks, and exact point locations of the below points.

THE SKILL

Key Acupressure/Acupuncture Points for Chronic Constipation (Please see my resource webpage for exact point locations and other constipation tips!) Press each of these points firmly for one to two minutes while breathing deeply for the most effectiveness. Pressing these points can potentially help anyone poop, whether it's your elderly mom or your toddler who can't seem to get things flowing.

Large Intestine 4 (LI 4): By gently pressing or massaging LI 4, you can help your body find some relief from chronic constipation. It's a small point, but it packs a big punch when it comes to getting things moving again! Located on the hand between the thumb and index finger, this point helps stimulate peristalsis and promotes bowel movement. This point helps get your digestive system moving, like hitting the start button on a sluggish engine. It encourages your intestines to move waste along more smoothly, making it easier to have a bowel movement. Sometimes, constipation happens because your body is holding on to too much tension. This point helps relax that tension that builds up from stress, anxiety, or just feeling physically tight.

Stomach 36 (ST 36): Located on the lower leg, this point strengthens the digestive system and boosts energy (qi), improving intestinal function. It's one of the most important points for improving digestion and overall health in Traditional Chinese Medicine (TCM). Besides boosting digestion, it helps kickstart your digestive system, making it more efficient at breaking down food and moving it through your intestines. When digestion is sluggish, it can cause constipation, but stimulating ST 36 helps get things back on track. Sometimes, constipation happens because your body is low on energy, or qi, which makes it hard for your intestines to push waste through. ST 36 strengthens your body's energy and helps give your digestive system the oomph it needs to move things along.

Furthermore, this point reduces bloating and discomfort. If you feel bloated or heavy when constipated, ST 36 can help relieve that uncomfortable feeling by supporting smoother digestion and reducing the buildup of gas and pressure. By stimulating ST 36, you're giving your digestive system the boost it needs to function better, making it a great point to target for chronic constipation relief. It's like giving your body a little extra fuel to get things moving!

San Jiao 6 (SJ 6): Located on the forearm, this point helps move qi and fluids, promoting better digestion and alleviating constipation. San Jiao 6 (SJ 6) is an acupuncture point located on the outer side of your forearm, about three finger widths above the wrist. It's a great point for helping with chronic constipation because it focuses on moving energy and fluids through your body. SJ 6 promotes bowel movements and is known for helping to get things moving in your digestive system. In school, we nicknamed this point the "fire in the hole" point because it is that effective at moving stool. Stimulating this point encourages the natural movement of your intestines, making it easier for you to have a bowel movement. If you're feeling bloated, tight, or uncomfortable due to constipation, SJ 6 helps relieve that stuck feeling by encouraging movement and reducing that sense of heaviness in your belly.

Overall, acupuncture helps treat chronic constipation by restoring balance in the body's energy flow, stimulating the digestive system, and addressing both the physical and emotional factors that may contribute to constipation. Regular acupuncture treatments, along with lifestyle and dietary changes, can lead to long-term relief from chronic constipation. If you'd like to dive in deeper and learn more about how acupuncture and Chinese medicine can help with constipation, I invite you to visit my resource page.

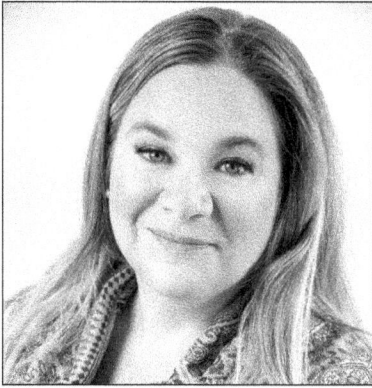

Dr. Heather Schuerlein is a Board-Certified Acupuncture Physician and Doctor of Acupuncture and Chinese Medicine. She completed her Doctoral degree at Pacific College of Oriental Medicine in New York, New York. She also holds two Master's degrees, one in Acupuncture and the other in Oriental Medicine (MSAOM) from Finger Lakes School of Acupuncture and Oriental Medicine at New York Chiropractic College in Seneca Falls, New York. Recently she obtained her fellowship in the Acupuncture Board of TCM reproductive medicine (ABORM, 2023). Her training encompasses Acupuncture, Chinese Herbal Medicine, Tuina (Chinese Medical massage), Qi gong, and Eastern dietary therapy. She also received training in Japanese acupuncture theory and techniques.

Dr. Heather's well-rounded experience includes but is not limited to providing care for various pain conditions, digestive and respiratory disorders, women's health, and sports related injury. She has worked in various settings including the Seneca Falls Health Center and the Veterans Affairs Hospital in Canandaigua, New York.

Heather is a member of the Phi Chi Omega honor society and studied abroad at the Zhejiang Provincial Hospital of Traditional Chinese Medicine in Hangzhou, China.

Connect with Dr. Heather:

Instagram: https://www.instagram.com/palmcoastacu/

Website: https://palmcoastacupuncture.com/

TikTok: https://www.tiktok.com/@drheatheracu

CHAPTER 15

YOU BECOME WHAT YOU SING ABOUT ALL DAY LONG

CRAFTING YOUR PERSONAL SONG FOR A LIFE OF RESONANCE AND MEANING

Michael MacDonald, iah.fit founder

Before I submitted this chapter to my publisher, I shared it with a select few, hoping to touch their hearts and inspire their spirits. Among them was my sister Shannon. She embraced the exercise wholeheartedly and stepped into the world I'd written about with open arms. When she sent back her personal statement, which I wasn't expecting, it was an aha moment for me. *Wow, this has impact*, I thought. *This can work.* And in fact, it just did. Her willingness to play the game with me, to dive into the depths of her own soul, moved me profoundly. It was a testament to the power of words and intention, and I knew I had to share her statement, which would then transform into her personal song within these pages.

"My word is my wand, and my feelings are my future. So, I use my words wisely and speak them with an open heart and loving mind."

~ Shannon MacDonald, Author, Healer

In a world overflowing with chaos and negativity—from media to relationships, politics to work—what if you could navigate it all with a personal anthem? Imagine a mantra that resonates with your deepest values and tunes you to your desired life. This isn't just a dream; it's a real possibility. As you explore these pages, you'll learn how to elevate your inner frequency, becoming unstoppable in any environment.

BUT FIRST-ENTRAINMENT

Have you ever noticed how one person's mood can change the energy of a room? That's not just a coincidence—it's entrainment. Entrainment is the phenomenon where independent rhythms—heartbeats, brainwaves, or the energy in a room—sync up, creating either harmony or disharmony.

As Eckhart Tolle writes in *The Power of Now:* "The energy field of a group of people will be strongly affected by the energy of the person who has the most intense presence." This is the essence of entrainment—the strongest rhythm or energy leads, pulling others into its flow, whether for positive or negative outcomes.

This explains how our internal frequency—shaped by our thoughts and words and amplified by our voice—can influence those around us. Your voice and presence can entrain others, creating either resonance or dissonance. The strongest frequency always leads, so the question is: *Will you be the tuner or the tuned?*

MY STORY

Isn't it strange how a song can seep into your skin, into your veins, like rain soaking into the Earth—slow and unnoticed—until it becomes part of you? I once believed that writing songs could heal me. If I gave my pain a melody, it would drift away. But it didn't. Instead, it burrowed deeper, each chorus binding it tighter.

I started out on Venice Beach, neon blue hair and all, writing raw, emotional songs—somewhere between Nirvana and Red Hot Chili Peppers. I thought clever hooks could lift the weight I carried. But catchy songs don't cure wounds—they trap you in them. My grief became a refrain, echoed back and amplified by others. Repetition doesn't heal; it deepens the groove.

Sorrow, when sung enough, becomes an identity. It hums between conversations and murmurs when no one's listening. It becomes a shadow stitched to your heels, following you even when you think you've outrun it. For years, that was my life—a chorus of shadows. Each note wound the thread tighter around the ache I was trying to escape.

PIVOTAL REALIZATION

One night, I sat at my desk, watching a glossy music video—*a billion views*, I thought. A billion souls entranced by this perfect song. The production was flawless, but beneath the beauty was simmering darkness—a story of violence, betrayal, and revenge. *What are we feeding people?* I wondered. *What are we teaching them without saying it outright?*

I glanced at the framed photos of my sons, Dylan (6) and Valentino (4)—so young, so impressionable. *What if they watched this? I thought. What would they learn without even realizing it?* My stomach tightened. They'd absorb the toxicity without knowing it, hypnotized by the beauty and glamour, learning distorted lessons about love, trust, and relationships.

Then it hit me: *Am I any different?* The realization hit like a spotlight to the eyes. My heart raced. I thought I was making art to heal, but I was just amplifying the pain.

My music wasn't freeing anyone—not me, not the people listening. I wasn't breaking chains; I forged new ones, entraining others into my own trauma with every catchy hook.

PERSONAL GROWTH JOURNEY

I spent years seeking personal growth and understanding, asking myself: *Who am I? Why am I here? Who is the "I" behind my words?* These questions led me through books, seminars, and countless conversations with experts. I became a lifelong student at what I call *YouTube University*—an education in passion and perseverance that no Ivy League could offer.

Every book and lecture opened new questions. But everything shifted when I read *Word I Am Word* by Paul Selig. He explores how words and intentions form the building blocks of life. One quote hit me deeply: "You are not only the speaker of your word, you are the vibration of the word that you speak." I realized that words don't just express thoughts—they shape reality.

After finishing the book, I couldn't sit still. I walked in circles, repeating to myself: *What words will I use to build my future? What do I want my life to look like?* Spelling is casting a spell. Are we not using our words as magic to shape our reality?

As Don Miguel Ruiz writes in *The Four Agreements*: "Be impeccable with your word. Speak with integrity. Say only what you mean. The word is the most powerful tool you have as a human; it is the tool of magic." That truth hit hard. Words, like spells, have the power to create or destroy, depending on how we use them.

MASTERING NLP AND TIME-LINE THERAPY

I was on a mission to master the power of words. I didn't just attend a few seminars—I dove headfirst into Neuro-Linguistic Programming, studying directly under Dr. Tad James, the godfather of Time-Line Therapy. Driven by an insatiable desire to understand the unconscious mind, I sought to break free from limiting patterns—and help others do the same.

As Dr. Tad James said, "The past does not equal the future unless you live there." By reprogramming my unconscious mind, I realized I could rewrite my story—and guide others to do the same.

I learned that words are the blueprint of our thoughts, shaping our reality. By tuning into the mind's rhythm, I shifted my own frequencies to create a life of purpose and power.

A MESSAGE TO SUPERSTARS

One evening, while searching for inspiration, I stumbled upon a TED Talk by Dr. Pennebaker titled *Your Words May Predict Your Future*. As I listened, goosebumps ran up my spine. *What if I were asked to speak on TED?* I wondered. *Do I have something valuable to say?*

In that moment, I knew I did. *Words are the key.* A rush of emotion followed, and I began writing—a letter to the world's superstars. *What do you want your legacy to be?* I urged them to distill their essence into a powerful statement—something worthy of their gravestone.

Imagine superstars around the world empowering their young audiences to become the greatest versions of themselves! That idea stirred my soul—the ripple effect of their influence could echo across generations.

Then, it hit me—suddenly and powerfully, like a door swinging open in my mind. *This isn't just for superstars.*

I froze, overwhelmed by the truth. I was so focused on those with celebrity and influence that I missed the most profound realization: *We are all alchemists.* Each of us holds the power to create the life we love through the magic of our words.

This wasn't just a thought—it was an awakening. Our words shape our reality, whether whispered in solitude or spoken on a stage. The message wasn't just for the superstars—it was for all of us.

We each have the ability to craft a personal song, tuning ourselves to a higher frequency and shaping our lives with purpose and intention. It's not about fame or fortune—it's about using the power of your word to manifest the life you truly desire.

Your word, backed by intention, is the key to everything.

CRAFTING A TRANSFORMATIVE SONG

Let's begin with me.

With my new guiding principle of *Tuned or Be Tuned*, I knew I had to craft my own powerful statement—a mantra to entrain myself into becoming all that I could be. Who am *I, really?* I thought. *What do I want my life to look like?* I wasn't just looking for words. I looked for something that grounded and inspired me, and carried me forward through life's storms. I wanted to be a great father, a husband, and a man worthy of respect. A man who leaves behind a legacy of inspiration and empowerment.

After long walks and moments of reflection, something finally emerged from my pen—a poem that felt like home:

I am worthy, I am light
Standing tall, reaching new height
Sun on my face, I embrace
The power within my sacred space
Boom, pow, I rise anew
In this world, my dreams pursue

It's interesting how I struggled with self-worth my entire life. As a child of divorce, I often felt unnoticed and replaceable—like I didn't matter. Those feelings lingered, shaping so many of my choices. But this poem—this was different. It wasn't just words on a page. It ignited something deep within me—a healing that reached down to the parts of myself I had long forgotten.

At first, I whispered it, unsure, testing the waters, feeling the power of each word as it left my lips. Each line felt like a stone dropped into a deep well, sending ripples through the layers of doubt and insecurity. Then I began to sing it. With each note, I felt the words taking root, vibrating through my core. *This is my song*, I thought. *This is what I will carry with me.*

For the first time, those words weren't just a fleeting affirmation. They were a declaration of my self-worth—etched into my soul, ready to guide me forward.

THE CALL TO ACTION

We learned that we live in a world shaped by vibrations and emotions, constantly influenced by the people and environments around us. But we don't have to be passive in this process. By tuning into our personal frequency—through our words and intentions—we can consciously shape the energy we emit and transform any situation.

You can be the strongest vibration in any room.

Writing down your passionate statement—whether it's a poem, a sentence, or even a bullet point—is the first important step. This act anchors your intention in the physical world. But the second, more powerful step is to bring that intention to life with your voice. When you speak or sing it, you're turning it into an audible frequency that entrains your entire nervous system—every cell and fiber of your being—into resonance with the power of your inspiration.

As sound healer Jonathan Goldman says in *The Humming Effect*: "Sound is a vibrational force that changes our reality. When we use our voice with intention, we send our desires out into the universe, vibrating through the ether of life."

Your word, amplified by your voice, becomes the dominant frequency in your life. This song isn't just a statement—it's a tool to navigate life's chaos with clarity and strength. Will you choose to become the tuner rather than be tuned?

The first step is answering these questions:

What defining statement is worthy of your gravestone?

Can you capture it in a single sentence?

This is your expression, your value to the world.

For example, *I am a beacon of light, harmonizing the world with my unwavering frequency of love and empowerment.*

So I ask you: *What song will you sing into existence?*

First...

THE SCIENCE OF INTENTION: WRITING TO SHAPE REALITY

"If you want to find the secrets of the universe, think in terms of energy, frequency, and vibration."

~Nikola Tesla

Writing down your intentions is more than self-expression—it's scientifically proven to make them more likely to manifest. This act engages the brain in a way that enhances memory and focus, turning abstract thoughts into tangible outcomes [2]. By transferring your ideas onto paper, you take the first step in aligning your desires with reality.

Quantum physics supports this, revealing that reality is shaped by frequency. Through wave-particle duality, we know particles exhibit wave-like behavior [4]. When your words and actions align with clear intention, you tune your personal frequency to resonate with the life you want. Your written song, charged with purpose, becomes a blueprint for transformation.

Neuroscience shows that repetition—whether through thought or action—reinforces neural pathways, carving new routes in your mind [7].

With each repetition of your mantra, you are rewiring your brain to move toward your desires.

THE SCIENCE OF AMPLIFICATION: SINGING AS AN INSTRUMENT OF CHANGE

"Quantum physics is the physics of possibilities, and it is where science and spirituality meet."

~ Dr. Amit Goswami

Dr. Goswami's words remind us that you merge science and spirit by vocalizing your song. Singing doesn't just connect with the world—it transforms it. You access the field of infinite possibilities through your voice and reshape your reality.

Quantum physics reveals that frequency shapes reality. You align your voice with universal frequencies by singing your intentions, harmonizing your inner and outer worlds [4]. Singing your song isn't merely an act of practice—it's an act of creation.

Sound directly affects your body and mind. Humming increases nitric oxide production, improving respiratory health [1], while singing stimulates the vagus nerve, easing anxiety and promoting emotional balance [3]. When you sing your personal song, you don't just express it—you embody it.

In Traditional Chinese Medicine (TCM), singing harmonizes the body's Qi, improving lung function, emotional release, and overall energy [5]. Sound shapes our energy field, creating balance and strength from within.

Let the tuning begin.

THE SKILL

Below is a guide to crafting your personal song—a statement you can carry within you, a rhythm that will shape your thoughts, your actions, and your reality. Each step is a thread waiting for you to weave into your own melody.

STEP 1: STEP INTO SILENCE

"In the silence of the mind, all answers lie."

~ Joel S. Goldsmith, *The Thunder of Silence*

Creation begins in silence—the pause before the first note, the breath before the leap. Disconnect from distractions. Listen to your breath, the gentle rhythm of your steps. This is your stage, your blank canvas. Softly ask: *What words do I want* to use to define my life, my future? *What story do I want 'spell' into existence?* Let silence cradle these questions. Answers will emerge in their own time, carried by the rhythm of your journey intent.

STEP 2: AUTOMATIC WRITING

"There is no doubt that writing automatically unlocks hidden layersof our consciousness."

~ Julia Cameron, *The Artist's Way*

Upon returning from silence, grab a blank page and let your thoughts flow. Write anything—nonsense, fears, dreams—without editing or overthinking. Let your words pour out like water over stones, smoothing as they go. Within this chaos, fragments of your true song will emerge, waiting to be discovered.

STEP 3: WHAT LIGHTS YOU UP?

"Pay attention to what lights you up. It's trying to lead you somewhere."

~ Danielle LaPorte, *The Fire Starter Sessions*

Review your writing and highlight the words and sentences that resonate profoundly and stir your spirit. These are the seeds of your personal song, the essence of your true self. Within these words lies your unbroken, rising potential.

STEP 4: SET IT TO RHYTHM

"Words are vibrations; let them resonate and fill the space with harmony."

~ John O'Donohue, *Anam Cara: A Book of Celtic Wisdom*

Speak your words aloud. Do they stumble or sing? Refine them until they flow effortlessly. This song is yours—sing it, hum it, whisper it. Let your voice shape your reality. Feel the vibration resonate through you, each syllable a note in your life's composition. The power lies in conviction, not just in words.

STEP 5: MAKE IT YOUR MANTRA

"With repetition, your words become your reality; your voice is the brush, painting the canvas of your life."

~ Marianne Williamson, *A Return to Love*

Repetition transforms. As you sing your song, it becomes part of you. Let it weave into your mornings, hum it in traffic, sing it in the shower. Gradually, your thoughts and actions will align with this new rhythm. You are tuning yourself to a new frequency, reshaping your life note by note.

FINAL CONCLUSION:

Your voice is more than sound—
it's the brush that paints your future.

Mastering your song isn't just an act—it's a way of living. It takes practice, like learning to ride a bike, but once you've mastered it, it becomes part of you. Your voice, powered by intention and purpose, can align your inner world with your desired life.

Imagine the doors that could open, the transformations that could unfold, when you fully embrace the magic of your words, amplified by your voice. The key to transformation has always been within you.

You are the one you've been waiting for.

YOUR PERSONAL SONG: NEXT STEPS

Over the past eight years, my journey—from an unaware singer-songwriter to an intentional song creator—reshaped my understanding of music, words, and frequency. What began as self-expression evolved into the realization that music, paired with clear intention, uplifts, energizes, and drives real change.

This insight inspired the creation of *iah.fit*, a platform designed to help you achieve vitality and balance through intentional music and Heart-Centered AI™. My personal transformation led to a groundbreaking tool to help you do the same.

At *iah.fit*, we've developed the first Resonance-Frequency Music™ generator. With the push of a button, you can turn your personal statement into a full-fledged song aligned with frequencies that elevate well-being and growth. Bring your song to life—own it, share it, and let it inspire both you and others on the journey to a life they love.

Embrace this experience and let your song tune your world.

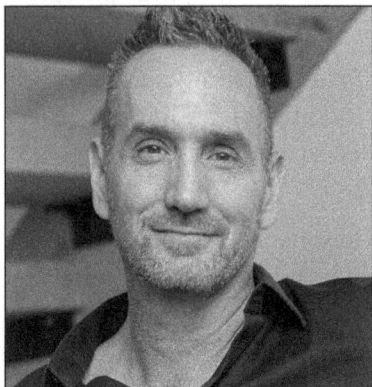

Michael MacDonald is a visionary leader, accomplished musician, and master Neuro-Linguistic Programming (NLP) trainer. Together with his wife, Francesca, he co-founded iah.fit. This revolutionary wellness platform merges ancient wisdom with cutting-edge technology to empower individuals on their path to optimal well-being. His pioneering work in Resonance Frequency Music™ and Sonic Supplements™ harnesses sound to align the body's energy fields, fostering vitality, balance, and peace.

As a former Marine, devoted father, and philanthropist, Michael is committed to building a legacy of wellness, strength, and empowerment for his sons, Dylan and Valentino, and for the wider world. He deeply believes in the transformative power of words and music to create profound change within individuals and the global community.

Connect with Michael:

https://iah.fit/michael-macdonald/

https://CraftMySong.ai/ to transform your statement into music with just a click.

LinkedIn: https://www.linkedin.com/in/mblu/

Resources
1. American Journal of Respiratory and Critical Care Medicine
2. Frontiers in Psychiatry
3. NIH–Heart Rate Variability
4. Physics World–Wave-Particle Duality and Quantum Mechanics
5. NIH–Effects of Singing on Respiratory Health
6. Physics World–Sound Manipulation
7. NIH–The Mind-Body Connection
8. NIH–The Impact of Singing on Emotional Health

REGULATION OF
THE NERVOUS SYSTEM

"Before the battle of the fist, comes the battle of the mind."

~ Master Shifu (Kung Fu Panda)

REGULATION OF THE NERVOUS SYSTEM:

AN OVERVIEW

What in the world is nervous system regulation? Essentially, it's your inner dialogue, the way you communicate with yourself to keep resilient and in balance. It's how you keep stress in check.

Throughout the chapters of this pillar, you'll hear more about an integral part of our physiology: The autonomic nervous system (ANS), which helps your body respond to stress when needed and relax when it's safe. The ANS affects every single part of our physiology. It oversees vital functions such as heart rate, digestion, metabolism, respiratory rate, and reproductive functions, all of which play crucial roles in maintaining our overall health and well-being. Your heart and your brain are the masters, and they keep everything working in sync.

While it's often easy to feel out of control, especially when there is a major stressor, or many minor ones at once, there are extremely powerful strategies you can utilize *on the spot* and *free of charge* to shift to a calmer, more productive state:

- **Your Breath**
  Intentionally using your breath to regain control of your physiological responses.

- **Your Emotions**
  Shifting your emotional state to a more positive/productive one.

- **Your Mindset**
  Reframing negative thoughts, and finding connection by staying mindful (being fully present and aware) of what's happening in the moment without judgment or distraction.

Developing skills in each will serve you lifelong, no matter your life stage or health circumstance, as you go through your day, as you quiet your mind at night, and as you connect with the people around you.

CHAPTER 16

BREATH:
YOUR ULTIMATE LIFE TOOL

UNLOCK LIFE'S POTENTIAL
WITH BREATH DESIGN

Stephen Dahmer, MD

MY STORY

I love to breathe. I also love to travel. On one memorable trip to the rock islands of Palau, an archipelago of over 500 islands in the Pacific Ocean, I was spearfishing with the son of the Chief when I nearly lost both loves. With hopes of impressing a new friend, I pushed myself to new depths, mesmerized by the underwater world in the blue waters of the Pacific. As I descended in pursuit of a captivating surgeonfish (a cerulean blue ray-finned fish), awe turned to angst when I gasped involuntarily, water flooding my mouth like liquid panic.

In a desperate struggle for air, I felt the deep fear of drowning and instinctively closed my mouth. I clamored to the surface of the water. As I broke the surface and gulped in life-giving oxygen, I experienced a profound revelation about the preciousness of each breath. This experience transformed my perspective and made me exceptionally mindful of how breath connects my body and mind.

Your breath is your life. Most of us get that—the literal part. Unfortunately, like me, we're reminded of it only when something completely takes our breath away.   I'm here to tell you that your breath is much more than life and death. I'm also asking you to please not wait for a shocking adventure like mine to learn about the ultimate life tool we regularly use but without proper awareness. To unlock this incredible gift, you must first move beyond the idea of breath being automatic and done without your input. The true magic of this remarkable tool comes alive when you start to shape your breath consciously.

Palau taught me the profound power of breath. My transition from believing that "breathing is necessary for my life" to "designing my breathing can impact my life positively" solidified during my one-year leave of absence from my medical school education.

I took a break from school because I was hungry for more out of life. During that year, I self-organized a new approach to my health education, one of the most transformative in my life as a young healer. I worked with primary care physicians, psychiatrists, medical anthropologists, herbalists, Umbandistas (practitioners of the Umbanda religion), and a renowned healer who taught breathwork as a tool to connect, calm, invigorate, restore, and empower. We practiced much of this breathwork education in extreme circumstances in Brazil's second-largest favela (low-income neighborhood), Pirambu. I witnessed directly how breath design was transformative in healing severe trauma, unlocking supernatural experiences, calming down panic, connecting more with others, and, just as important, simply feeling better. One of my most vivid memories was in a *Casa de Caboclo*, a single room that served as a refuge space and was filled with a rainbow of paintings, statues of *orixas* (spiritual entities), altars covered with candles, drumming in the background, and a haze of sweet-smelling incense.

Breath is the best regulator of stress and health; you have minute-to-minute access to and control over it. I want to help you design your breath to optimize your life.

As a practicing physician, I've observed the transformative power of breath for decades. During those years, I dedicated myself to exploring the depths of this ancient wisdom, teaching countless patients the simple yet profound practice of conscious breathing. And I witnessed firsthand the astonishing results: children with asthma gaining more control over their breath, patients during a panic attack seeing their breath as an anchor to hold and regain their balance, numerous people overwhelmed with stress, reporting back the power of this simple tool in regaining control over their nervous system. So many of my patients have reported reduced stress, increased calm, improved sleep, and enhanced physical resilience in the face of illness. More important than all that is self-empowerment. Your breath empowers you with the most excellent tool on your health journey.

Have you ever felt like you're constantly on high alert? We far too often race through our day with a sense of urgency, like the world is moving so quickly that we can barely keep up. When we feel like this, our body's default mode is often stuck in fight or flight, courtesy of the sympathetic nervous system (SNS). This robust response is designed to help us react quickly to threats, but when triggered too frequently, it can leave us feeling frazzled and exhausted. Luckily, nature's intelligence built in a counterbalance: the parasympathetic nervous system (PNS), often referred to as "rest and digest" mode. This calming force built into our nervous system helps our body relax, repair, and rejuvenate—cue your deeper breathing, slower heart rate, and a sense of calm clarity. Modern life encourages many of us to spend way too much time in sympathetic overdrive and not enough in parasympathetic tranquility. Again, with regular practice of simple techniques like conscious breathing, we shift our nervous system into PNS mode, where we tap into the body's innate ability to heal, recharge, and find peace amidst life's stressors.

Yet, despite its life-changing potential, many people underestimate the power of breath, viewing it as a mere new age "quick fix" or a fleeting distraction from their daily worries. I implore you: don't make this mistake! Take up the practice of conscious breathing wholeheartedly, with the same level of commitment and dedication that you would any critical aspect of your life.

In the stillness and calm of each breath lies a deep wellspring of resilience, waiting to be tapped—precisely this inner strength that can illuminate even the darkest moments on our life journey. Tools are mostly helpful but can also cause harm (we've all cut ourselves with a knife or even hit a finger with a hammer). Use this versatile tool to your advantage. Do not delay another minute. One of the most significant health tools ever created is your breath, and if you aren't harnessing the power of this tool, you're missing out.

THE SKILL

The awareness we give our breath and how we design our life by using breath can change how we live. It's said that the river can change its course if you move the rocks. Our breath is the rocks that direct the river of our life. I encourage you to set the rocks of breath intentionally and with awareness.

The most potent breathing exercise I have learned is the 4-7-8 breathing exercise, also known as the *Relaxation Breath*. I've practiced it for over 30 years and learned it from Dr. Andrew Weil, a mentor, a world-renowned physician, and a pioneer in integrative medicine. Integrative medicine is a healing-oriented healthcare approach encompassing body, mind, and spirit. He popularized this breathing technique, which calms the nervous system, reduces stress, and promotes relaxation. By manipulating the breath in a specific pattern, you can directly influence your brain's response to stress and anxiety.

How to Practice the 4-7-8 Breathing Exercise

Please put everything down. Put yourself in the right state of mind. Come and join me completely in this transformative experience. To begin, find a quiet and comfortable place to sit or lie down, ideally with your back supported. Close your eyes and take a moment just to be.

1. The T-Tap: Begin by touching the tip of your tongue to the roof of your mouth, just behind your top teeth. Doing so will help you breathe more slowly and deliberately.

2. Inhale (4 counts): Inhale through your nose for a count of four. Feel the breath fill your lungs fully without trying to control its depth or speed.

3. Hold (7 counts): Hold your breath for a count of seven. This allows you to feel a slight increase in carbon dioxide levels, which signals your brain that you are relaxed.

4. Exhale (8 counts): Exhale through your mouth audibly for a count of eight. I find it very powerful to use my mind's eye to release tension or thoughts as I exhale, picturing them leaving my body as I breathe.

THE KEY ELEMENTS

- Touching the tip of your tongue to the roof of your mouth helps slow down your breathing, making it more meditative and calming. It also relaxes your jaw and slows your heart rate—a remarkable impact for such a simple gesture.

- The specific ratio of inhaling (4 counts) to holding (7 counts) to exhaling (8 counts) is important to induce a state of relaxation. This balance affects the brain's response to stress hormones like cortisol. I'm often asked why there is a specific ratio of 4:7:8. The seven-second hold may help increase CO_2 levels in the blood, which can have a calming effect on the nervous system. The extended eight-second exhale likely activates the parasympathetic nervous system, further promoting relaxation and reducing stress. I strive to honor and preserve the oral traditions and practices passed down to me, as they have been validated and enriched through generations of wisdom and experience.

- Engaging the diaphragm during breathing is crucial to maximize the benefits of any breathwork. By activating this dome-shaped muscle at the base of your lungs, you can increase lung capacity, improve oxygen exchange, and stimulate the vagus nerve, which triggers the body's relaxation response.

- To engage your diaphragm in breathing, place one hand on your chest and the other on your belly, just below your rib cage. As you inhale through your nose, focus on pushing your belly outward while keeping your chest relatively still. This conscious effort to expand your abdomen rather than your chest ensures you use your diaphragm effectively for deeper, more efficient breaths.

- As you practice this technique regularly, your body responds by releasing physical tension, reducing your heart rate, and calming your mind, body, and spirit.

You can easily find many videos of Dr. Weil instructing the 4-7-8 breathing exercises online. This is one of my favorites: https://bit.ly/drweil478

I encourage you to watch and learn from Dr. Weil himself. You can also find further instructions on diaphragm breathing and what to do if the exercise feels challenging at first on the internet: https://bit.ly/drweildiaphragm

Dr. Weil has written extensively about the benefits of breathwork in his books and online courses. His approach to integrative medicine emphasizes the importance of mindfulness, self-awareness, and natural healing methods. By learning this simple yet powerful breathing technique, you can tap into the wisdom of centuries-old breathing practices while benefiting from a modern scientific understanding of stress and its impact on your health.

Please remember that consistent practice will help you experience the full benefits of the 4-7-8 breathing exercise. The 4-7-8 is not a "one and done" exercise but a regular ritual that strengthens the more you practice. Be sure to incorporate it into your routine at least twice daily. I find it to be even more powerful if you practice when you are *not* experiencing stress or anxiety. The work you put into it now will be well worth its while and significantly impact your nervous system when needed in the future.

As you work to design your breath, it will eventually highlight the tremendous impact it has on life and health during a highly stressful or anxious situation. When faced with intense stress or anxiety, many people experience rapid, shallow breathing that, if left unchecked, can exacerbate feelings of panic. When we do this, we are hitting our own thumb with the hammer! By consciously slowing and deepening the breath in these moments, you can trigger the body's relaxation response and dramatically shift the course of your physiological and psychological state.

For example, imagine you're about to give an important presentation or performance, and just before the event, you feel incredibly nervous. Your heart is racing, your palms are sweaty, and your thoughts are scattered. By taking a few minutes to practice slow, deep 4-7-8 breathing, you can:

- Interrupt the cycle of anxious thoughts
- Lower your heart rate and blood pressure
- Reduce levels of stress hormones like cortisol
- Increase oxygen flow to your brain and improve mental clarity
- Stimulate the nervous system

Within just a few minutes of controlled breathing, you may find your anxiety has decreased significantly. Your mind feels clearer, your body more relaxed, and you can approach the presentation more calmly and confidently.

This tangible shift from a state of stress to one of relative ease through the simple act of breathing illustrates the profound connection between breath, mind, and body. It demonstrates how breath can be a powerful tool for self-regulation and wellbeing that we always carry with us. Additionally, it's a tool you have inside that goes everywhere with you. No tool belt required! No pharmacy required! And it's free to use anytime! These advantages makes breathing a remarkable tool for our health.

Breath is a powerful anchor to the present moment, a reminder of stillness, presence, and being. Recognizing your breath as a tool for stillness and presence can cultivate a more profound sense of being in each moment. Many cultures have long recognized breathing as vital for health and spirituality. Modern research continues to validate breathwork's wide-ranging benefits for physical and mental health. The most convincing research will be your own; please try this out and try it often. I'm confident you'll be delighted with the results of your rediscovered, versatile health tool.

While the 4-7-8 is my preferred choice, remember that many tools and techniques exist to help you harness the transformative power of your breath. Find the one that best works for you! Ideally, it should be one that you look forward to and enjoy practicing. My esteemed colleagues have expanded on this crucial concept in some of our subsequent chapters. Breathe easy; the most important thing is finding what works best through practice and experimentation. See your life as a river and use your breath to place the stones that will shape its flow, guiding your health and well-being in a positive direction.

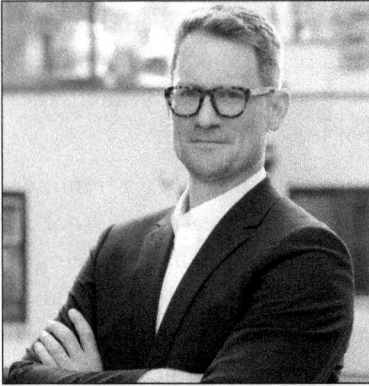

As Director of the Andrew Weil Center for Integrative Medicine (AWCIM), **Dr. Stephen Dahmer** is a champion for integrative medicine and an integral force in transforming modern healthcare. As a cornerstone of the University of Arizona, AWCIM empowers thousands of healthcare practitioners to deliver evidence-based, integrative care that profoundly impacts lives. In his dual role as director and practicing physician, Dr. Dahmer is unwavering in his commitment to pioneering new standards in compassionate, patient-centered care through research, teaching, and clinical practice.

Dr. Dahmer's dedication to reshaping healthcare has taken him across the globe, from the favelas of Brazil and the Maori iwi communities in New Zealand to service as a hospitalist in the Navajo Nation in Arizona.

With a medical degree from the University of Wisconsin-Madison and fellowship training in Integrative Family Medicine at AWCIM, his distinguished career has included academic and clinical roles at institutions such as Mount Sinai School of Medicine and Albert Einstein College of Medicine.

Throughout his journey, Dr. Dahmer has held influential positions, including Lead Physician at Iora Health, Chief Medical Officer at Goodness Growth, and founding Primary Care Physician at Sana Care. His research focuses on unlocking the real-world outcomes of integrative therapies and the healing potential of medicinal plants, driving forward a vision of healthcare that nurtures and inspires practitioners and patients alike.

Connect with Dr. Stephen Dahmer:

Website: www.stephendahmermd.com

Andrew Weil Center for Integrative Medicine: https://awcim.arizona.edu/

LinkedIn: www.linkedin.com/in/stephendahmermd

Instagram: https://www.instagram.com/stephendahmermd/

CHAPTER 17

CHAOS TO CALM

THE HEART IS THE WAY

Patrick J. Nardulli, USN (Ret),
Resilience & Human Performance Expert

MY STORY

I was her hero until the day I lost my Dad superpower.

As I stood there, I watched my six-year-old daughter unravel before my eyes, her small frame trembling with an intensity that seemed to shake the very air around us. Her eyes, usually so bright and full of curiosity, were wide with terror, darting around the room as if searching for an escape from an invisible threat. Her face was flushed, a deep crimson spreading across her cheeks, and her breaths came in ragged, shallow gasps that seemed to echo in the silence of the room.

Her hands were clenched into tight fists at her sides, knuckles white with the strain, and her shoulders were hunched as if she were trying to make herself smaller, to disappear from whatever caused her such distress. Her whole body seemed to vibrate with a chaotic energy, a physical manifestation of the turmoil unfolding inside her mind.

In that moment, I felt a profound sense of helplessness wash over me; a heavy weight settled in my chest. I wanted nothing more than to reach out and pull her into my arms, to shield her from whatever storm was swirling inside her. But I knew my touch might only add to her overwhelm and push her further into the chaos.

"Sweetheart," I said softly, my voice steady and calm despite the turmoil I felt inside. "I'm here. You're safe. Just breathe with me, okay? In and out, nice and slow."

I watched as she struggled to follow my words, her breaths still coming in quick, uneven bursts. My heart ached with the desire to take away her pain, to make everything better with a simple hug or whispered reassurance. But all I could do was stand there, grounded and present, offering her the stability she so desperately needed.

"It's okay to feel scared," I continued, keeping my voice low and soothing. "I'm right here with you. You're not alone."

As I spoke, I focused on my own breathing, drawing in deep, steady breaths in the hope that she might mirror my calm. I felt the tension in my own body, the instinctive urge to fix, protect, and make everything right. But I knew this was her journey, her moment to navigate, and all I could do was be there, a steady presence in the storm.

In that moment, I understood the depth of my love for her—the fierce, unwavering commitment to stand by her side no matter what. And though I felt helpless, I also felt a quiet strength, a certainty that together, we'd weather this storm and emerge stronger on the other side—and we did, her breaths eventually found a steady rhythm, her fists unclenched, and her small frame leaned into me, seeking comfort as the storm inside her finally began to calm.

I knew then that I never again wanted her to feel that level of internal chaos, fear, or helplessness.

In the quiet moments after witnessing my daughter's emotional meltdown, I reflected deeply on the experience. Her terror-laden eyes mirrored a chaos I recognized all too well from my own life—chaos I had seen during multiple military deployments overseas, in the eyes of junior sailors, Marines, and even the seasoned faces of senior leadership. The battlefield, with its relentless demands, often left us all teetering on the edge of our emotional limits. The chaos of war echoed the chaos I saw in my daughter, serving as a stark reminder of the universal struggle with vulnerability, overwhelm, and emotional regulation.

This marked a profound awakening for me, igniting a passion to understand and master the nervous system—the very system that underlies these experiences.

That night, as I lay awake replaying the scene in my mind, I realized I needed to understand what had happened to my daughter. I delved into the **physiology of stress** (what happens in our body and brain before, during, and after a stressful event), **emotional regulation** (the ability to recognize and shift how we feel), and the intricacies of the **autonomic nervous system** (the key governor of our body's automatic processes), driven by a desire to help her—and others like her—find peace amidst the storm.

Over the years (she's now 25), I've had the privilege of turning what I've learned into actionable tools that I've empowered my daughter with, as well as those I train and coach daily—military personnel, first responders, caregivers and individuals navigating their own inner battles. I teach those in my care how to master their own nervous systems and find resilience in the face of life's chaos.

THE SKILL

Transitioning from personal narrative to the scientific exploration of nervous system regulation, it's essential to **recognize the profound connection between our emotional experiences and physiological responses.**

The story of my daughter's dysregulation serves as a poignant reminder of how deeply intertwined our emotions are with the autonomic nervous system (ANS) and heart rhythms, such as heart rate variability (HRV). These physiological markers not only reflect our current state of well-being and resilience but also offer insights into our capacity for emotional regulation and mental flexibility.

Emotions can be understood as "Energy in Motion". It's the physiology that we feel as our brain interprets and reacts to thoughts, experiences, and external events.

Emotional Regulation is the ability to recognize, understand and manage our body's emotional responses effectively. It means leveraging emotions as information and making intentional decisions about how to respond.

Our Autonomic Nervous System (ANS) governs 90% of our body's "automatic" internal functions, such as heart rate, breathing, digestion, and more.

Heart Rate Variability (HRV) is the most effective measure of our nervous system's resilience and adaptability. HRV reflects the variation in time between heartbeats, indicating how well our body can respond to stress and return to a balanced baseline.

Understanding a little bit of the science behind these processes, and how they interconnect empowers us to transform personal experiences of chaos into opportunities for coherence and growth.

BIOFEEDBACK—THE WINDOW INTO OUR NERVOUS SYSTEM

Have you ever wondered how we can actually "see" what's happening inside our bodies in real time? That's where biofeedback comes in—a fascinating way to observe our body's inner workings. Imagine having a special mirror that reflects not just our outward appearance but our inner body's signals, like heart rate or muscle tension, offering insights into how our mind and body work together.

What is biofeedback and why is it important?

Simply said, biofeedback is feedback about our biology.

Biofeedback commonly utilizes tech to provide *real-time* physiological feedback, enabling us to gain greater awareness and control over our body's processes.

It's like having a two-way conversation with our body, where technology translates physiological signals into actionable insights about how the body responds and recovers from stress. Think of it as a personal coach that guides us to better health and well-being by showing you how our body reacts to different situations.

Equipping both adults and children alike with biofeedback can teach us valuable skills for managing stress and emotions, while enhancing performance. There are many forms and all aim to help us become more aware of our body's signals, most notably from the state of the autonomic nervous system, and how to respond to them.

The autonomic nervous system is the silent conductor orchestrating the symphony of our body's involuntary functions and our heart rhythms. Its two main components -the sympathetic and parasympathetic branches -work collaboratively to keep our body in balance and in sync.

Various technologies can tell us if our ANS physiology is operating in a balanced state. We'll link to some in our resources. But for this chapter, we'll give you a sneak peek of simple tactics that you can use, without technology, to have greater control over your body's automatic or natural stress responses—to "feel" the state of your body and adjust it through focused attention.

STEP-BY-STEP EXERCISE: CONNECTING TO OUR ANS THROUGH THE RHYTHM OF THE HEART

Have you ever thought about how something as simple as your breath can directly influence the rhythm of your heart?

Today, we're diving into the fascinating connection between our breath, a focus on our heart, and how this intentional action can influence our heart's rhythm.

1. **Find a Comfortable Position:** Sit up straight and relax your shoulders. You can close your eyes if that helps you focus.

2. **Locate Your Pulse:** Place the index and middle fingers of one hand gently on the wrist of your opposite hand. Feel for your pulse on the inner side of your wrist, right below the base of your thumb.

3. **Observe Your Heartbeat:** Take a moment to simply observe your heartbeat. Notice its rhythm and pace. This is your baseline heart rate.

4. **Connect with Your Breath:** Inhale slowly and deeply through your nose. As you do this, feel the expansion of your chest and abdomen. *Slowly* exhale through your mouth, maintaining a smooth and controlled breath.

5. **Notice Changes and Reflect:** While continuing to breathe in this way, pay attention to the pulse on your wrist. Do you notice any changes in its rhythm or intensity as you breathe in and out? You might feel your heart rate *quicken* on the inhale… and *slow* on the exhale. This subtle variation—known as heart rate variability (HRV)—is a natural, adaptive response managed by your autonomic nervous system (ANS).

The autonomic nervous system (ANS) manages heart rate variability (HRV) through its two branches: the sympathetic and parasympathetic nervous systems. The sympathetic branch activates the "fight or flight" response, **increasing heart rate during inhalation.** Conversely, the parasympathetic branch promotes "rest and digest," **slowing the heart rate during exhalation.** This dynamic balance between the two branches allows the body to adapt to stress and maintain emotional regulation, ensuring stability and resilience.

By practicing this simple awareness exercise, you can tap into the fascinating interplay between two key physiological processes- your breath and heart rhythm, and deepen your understanding of HRV, one of the most reliable indicators of health, well-being, self-regulation, and performance. Consistently tuning into these rhythms can help promote a balanced and resilient nervous system.

HEART RATE VARIABILITY (HRV)—THE RHYTHM OF RESILIENCE

Have you ever thought about how your heart beats? Most of us imagine it as a steady drumbeat, right? But here's a fascinating fact: in a healthy, resilient person, the time between each heartbeat fluctuates slightly. This variation is known as heart rate variability or HRV.

So, what exactly is HRV?

Heart Rate Variability (HRV) reflects the balance and synchronization between the sympathetic and parasympathetic branches of the autonomic nervous system.

While heart rate tells us how many times our heart beats per minute, HRV measures the changes in time between those beats. *Imagine it like this:* instead of a metronome ticking at a constant pace, your heart rhythm is more like a dance, speeding up and slowing down as needed, meeting the demands of your day.

Why does this matter?

A high HRV is like having a heart and nervous system that are ready for anything. Whether you're running to catch a bus, helping a child with a challenging task or unwinding after a demanding day, your body can quickly shift between peak performance and recovery.

It's the dynamic balance between the intensity of "fight or flight" and the restorative power of "rest and recovery," allowing you to stay resilient, perform at your best, and bounce back better.

Baseline HRV: A measurement of personal adaptability and resilience of our nervous system. Individualized to each person serves as a starting point for improvement through intentional lifestyle practices.

Higher HRV: Reflects a high level of nervous system flexibility and resilience; indicates the ability to adapt more effectively to stress.

Lower HRV: Suggest a less flexible and resilient nervous system, making it harder to adapt to life's demands.

Here's the good news—you can boost your HRV! In addition to foundational lifestyle strategies, techniques like heart-focused breathing and using biofeedback technology not only help you track, but also empower you to actively improve it. It's all about implementing these practices into your daily routine to enhance your heart's adaptability, promote stress resilience, and better respond to life's challenges.

So, next time you feel your heart racing or slowing down, remember—it's not just a beat; it's a conversation between your heart and your body, adapting to whatever life throws your way.

COHERENCE—THE OPTIMAL STATE OF BEING

Understanding the link between heart rhythms, particularly Heart Rate Variability (HRV) and Emotions offers valuable insights into nervous system regulation and overall well-being. **By focusing on our heart and tuning into our body's emotional state, we can apply simple techniques to shift our heart rhythms into an optimal state of what scientists call *Physiological Coherence,*** where the heart and brain synchronize, leading to emotional stability and physiological efficiency. The coherence of our heart's rhythm—*heart rhythm coherence*— is a direct reflection of this.

Imagine being able to transform a moment of mental, emotional, and physiological chaos into one of calm and clarity with just a few intentional breaths. Let's explore another practical exercise that will guide you in harnessing the power of your heart rhythms to achieve this state of coherence, transforming chaos into calm by tuning in and shifting our state.

STEP-BY-STEP EXERCISE: TUNE IN AND SHIFT YOUR HEART RHYTHMS

Step 1: Grounding Presence

- **Action:** Find a quiet space where you can sit comfortably with your feet flat on the ground. Close your eyes and take a deep breath, feeling the connection between your body and the earth.

- **Purpose:** Grounding yourself physically helps anchor your mind and body, creating a stable foundation for emotional balance.

Step 2: Tune into your Current State

- **Action:** Ask yourself, "What am I feeling in my body right now?" Observe without judgment—do you feel tension, restlessness, calm, joy, or something else? Allow yourself to name the emotion or sensation you're experiencing.

- **Purpose:** Recognizing your current emotional and physiological state is the first step in understanding their impact on your nervous system and heart rhythms, and towards making an intentional shift to a more renewing state.

Step 3: Heart-Focused Breathing™

- **Action:** Close your eyes or gaze down at a 45-degree angle. Focus your attention in the area of your heart. Imagine your breath flowing in and out of your heart, breathing a little slower and deeper than usual. (You can even place your hand or both hands on your heart to bring your attention there). Find an easy rhythm that's comfortable. (*adapted from HeartMath™ Institute*)

- **Purpose:** Focusing on the area of the heart gets us out of our head and into our body, neutralizing the intensity of an emotional reaction. It also *begins* the shift of our heart rhythm to a more physiologically coherent state between the body and mind..

Step 4: Positive Emotion Activation

- **Action:** As you continue focusing on the area of your heart, think of someone, something, or an experience in your life that evokes a positive emotion, such as appreciation, care, compassion, gratitude, love, or joy. Allow yourself to fully experience this emotion.

- **Purpose:** Activating positive emotions creates an impactful shift in your emotional state and heart rhythms, which moves into a renewed, sustainable state. It also has a positive carryover effect on hormones like oxytocin, serotonin, and DHEA, often referred to as the vitality hormone.

  Suggestion: Maintain this practice for 5–10 minutes. This, combined with the activation of positive emotions, is crucial for achieving optimal heart rhythm coherence.

  The American Journal of Cardiology published research conducted at the HeartMath™ Research Institute that showed how emotional states are reflected in the heart rhythm patterns.

Step 5: Coherence Reflection

- **Action:** After a few minutes of breathing with a focus on the area of the heart and positive emotion activation, take a moment to reflect on any changes in your emotional and physical state.

- **Purpose:** Reflection helps reinforce the connection between your mental, emotional, and physical state.

Step 6: Integration and Intention

- **Action:** Set an intention to carry this sense of coherence and composure into your daily activities. Visualize yourself responding to future challenges with the same composure and clarity.

- **Purpose:** Intention-setting solidifies the practice, empowering you to access heart rhythm coherence whenever needed.

By incorporating this practice into your routine and carrying the sense of coherence into your daily life, you gain the tools to respond to stress with clarity and composure. This is the power of heart rhythm coherence— learning to shift into coherence not only benefits your entire body, it also enhances emotional resilience, improves cognitive performance, increases energy, and fosters a state of flow and inner ease.

PRACTICAL STRATEGIES FOR EVERYDAY CHALLENGES:

Life is full of moments that test our energy, focus, and resilience. These practical tools will help you prepare for challenges, navigate difficult situations, and recover with renewed strength and energy, ensuring you're always ready for what's next.

1. **Preparing for a Stressful Situation:** Anticipate upcoming events, situations or interactions and use this practice beforehand to center yourself, save energy, and boost performance.

2. **During a Challenging Moment:** Notice if you're reacting impulsively, pause, assess your state, and shift as needed to respond calmly and intentionally.

3. **Recovering After Stress:** Reflect on the event's impact; use this coherence practice to restore your energy and rebuild resilience for your next challenge.

Reflecting on my journey, from the challenges of military deployments to the tender moments with my daughter, I've come to understand the profound connection between our emotional experiences and physiological responses.

As a father, former military medical provider, and human resiliency coach, I've witnessed firsthand the transformative power of mastering the rhythms of the heart. The tools in this chapter will allow you and the children in your care to start doing so too.

Imagine your child learning to calm their racing heart before a big test or relaxing their tense muscles after a long day — when adults learn and practice these skills, they become invaluable role models for children, instilling lifelong skills that empower them to navigate their own lives with resilience and confidence, using the science and wisdom of the heart.

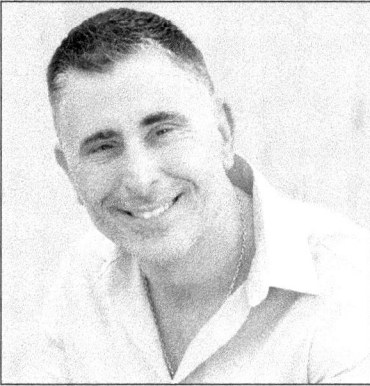

Patrick J. Nardulli, USN (Ret.), is a 20-year Navy veteran and a leading authority in human performance and resilience-building. He consults for military, first responder agencies, veteran-serving non-profits, and research groups, delivering evidence-based strategies to foster individual and organizational resilience.

Central to Patrick's work, he is driven by his passion for unlocking human potential, where he draws on the wealth of science and research in human performance optimization.

Patrick leverages his deep understanding of the mind-body connection, drawing on insights from extensive research in health, neuroscience, psychophysiology, and sleep science, emphasizing the power and science of the heart, underscoring the heart's crucial role in achieving lasting health and peak performance. He is trained in Mind-Body Mental Fitness (MBMF) and Combat and Operational Stress Control (COSC), and he holds multiple certifications from the HeartMath Institute.

When he's not busy unlocking human potential, Patrick loves diving into a good book or penning his thoughts. He's a fan of picking up and swinging heavy things—kettlebells, anyone?—and never misses a chance to break a sweat or test his mental and emotional endurance with a hot yoga session, a cold plunge, or the latest science-backed longevity hack.

Weekends are for adventure, so you'll find Patrick hiking, swimming, or cycling, all while soaking up community vibes and cultural experiences. Above all, Patrick cherishes time spent with his family, who are his greatest source of inspiration and support.

Connect with Patrick Nardulli:

Website: www.patricknardulli.com

Email: patrick@patricknardulli.com

LinkedIn: https://www.linkedin.com/in/patrick-nardulli-17662827/

Facebook: https://www.facebook.com/PatrickNardulliCoaching

CHAPTER 18

GET OUT OF THE GLASS PRISON

THE ULTIMATE SOLUTION TO HAPPINESS!

Philippe Brouillard, MBA, PhD cand. Quantum Science

MY STORY

From a young age, I felt disconnected and out of place. School teachings didn't resonate with me, and I couldn't see their relevance to real life. By 14, I was ready to leave it all behind, feeling unmotivated and detached from society's path.

I remember being called into the principal's office with my parents, and the school's director said, "You're the third-best student in your entrance exams." I stared blankly. *So what?* Despite excelling academically, school felt meaningless. I completed high school out of obligation, not passion. In pre-university, I rebelled, skipping classes and letting my grades slip. Sports became my escape, and I ranked 21st in Canada for freestyle skiing. It gave me joy and a sense of belonging.

However, my passion waned as the focus shifted to technicalities over the freedom and creativity of the jumps I loved. So, I quit. I was then drawn to functional medicine, inspired by my father, a medical doctor. I attempted to return to academia and applied to medical school. I had high hopes but faced rejection due to my unconventional path.

Shifting my focus to entrepreneurship, I pursued an MBA and, together with my wife, Natasha Azrak, built a successful health clinic, generating over $1.2 million yearly. On the surface, I was thriving. We built something successful and impactful. Yet inside, I was trapped in what I now call my glass prison. I was constantly doing, helping more people, achieving more, and building more systems, but it wasn't aligned with my inner being. I didn't even know what that truth was at the time.

Then we finally took a three-week vacation for the first time. It was in Bali and there my wife kept on saying, "I've never seen so much light in your eyes." It made me realize I was looking for something deeper.

I fell upon a doctorate in quantum science. Then, it was as if everything aligned.

My wife was also in the glass prison. She loved what she did and the impact. We were together for 12 years, and both wanted children, but if she went on maternity leave, eight employees would be out of a job since everything relied on her seeing and servicing our clients.

One day, she said, "That's it, I can't keep on putting my personal life on pause; we're stopping our clinical programs." You have to understand that these programs were bringing in 90% of our revenue.

I replied: "Wait a second, we both built this business; I have a say in this as well."

And then she said this simple phrase: "But you want out as well." She continued: "Imagine, you'll be free to do your quantum doctorate, even go on your Nepal trip you've always wanted to do!"

Everything aligned beautifully for our employees as well. Sometimes, life is just waiting for you to take the leap into what's more meaningful, for you to realize it's actually better for everyone.

So, I immersed myself full-time in my doctorate in quantum science, and for the first time, I started to understand the deeper questions that had plagued me since childhood.

Quantum science provided me with a framework to make sense of my journey. It wasn't just about success or recognition. It was about existence itself—why we are here and how we can align with our true purpose. **I realized I was stuck in the "school of work" (doing) when I should've been in the "school of life" (being).** Through quantum physics, I finally got answers for my Cartesian (scientific proof), pragmatic (need for being applicable) brain.

It showed me the science and proof that the universe isn't built on separation but on interconnectedness and energy.

For example, in the mind-blowing study by Jacobo Grinberg-Zylberbaum (1982), two people meditated together and then were separated. When lights were flashed in one's eyes, the other's brain, in a different room, mirrored the activity. This suggests instant brain communication (quantum entanglement), proving a deep, non-physical interconnection between us all.

Imagine being able to connect and positively influence the brain of another person in another part of the world, whether it's your child or a loved one.

Once you understand that everything is connected, your perception of your glass prison shatters. I realized my limits were a construct of my old way of thinking, a way of life based on external achievements and doing more instead of understanding the power of being. And I paid the cost for that.

Embracing quantum reality revealed that true freedom and happiness aren't tied to achievements but aligning with the universe's energy. Many are trapped in a cycle of "doing" for happiness, yet it's found in "being." I wasn't stuck after all. I simply viewed the world through the wrong lens. This is the lesson I wish to share.

THE SKILL

UNDERSTANDING TRUE HAPPINESS THROUGH QUANTUM CONSCIOUSNESS

So, what does this mean for you?

When you understand the difference between classical physics and quantum physics, you can break free from the glass prison and start to live a happier, stress-free life.

For a long time, people thought the world worked in a predictable, straight-line way. This idea came from classical (Newtonian) physics, which said that things follow clear rules, like cause and effect. But **quantum physics** changed everything. It showed us that everything is made of tiny particles of energy, like atoms and electrons, and that these particles don't always act in predictable ways.

At this tiny level, the world isn't fixed or solid. Instead, it's full of possibilities. **Dr. Amit Goswami**, a pioneer in the field of quantum consciousness and my doctorate mentor, explains that reality is like a "field of possibilities," always changing and shaped by our thoughts and choices. This means that our consciousness—the way we think and feel—can influence what happens around us.

In an experiment done in space, scientists noticed that particles changed their behavior just by being observed. This is called the **observer effect**. It means that by simply watching, we affect how things happen. This effect was first discovered in a famous experiment called the **double-slit experiment**, which showed that particles can act like waves or particles depending on whether they're being observed.

What does this all mean? It means that **reality isn't just happening to us**—we play a part in shaping it with the thoughts and choices we make, even if we're not consciously aware of it. Quantum experiments like these show that our reality isn't set in stone but is fluid and responds to our actions and awareness.

This understanding is what allows us to break free from the glass prison. When we view the world through a quantum lens, we see that the limitations we've imposed on ourselves—our sense of lack, our fears, our insecurities—are illusions. They're not real. They're simply products of the old way of thinking, rooted in the material, classical Newtonian view of reality. Just like I used to think I had no other way than to be in the glass prison of my past successful and impactful clinic.

THE BIGGEST TRAP

In our modern world, most of us operate from the mindset of listing everything we have to *do* and then going for it. We're constantly trying to achieve, acquire, and accumulate security. We think that by **doing** more, we will eventually have enough to be happy. It's the "Do, Have, Be" model (a linear, cause-and-effect model like classical physics).

This approach to life is deeply flawed because it places happiness as a future destination (separate from us), something to be pursued rather than experienced in the present. This leads to the **Hedonic Treadmill**—the more we chase pleasure and external success, the more it eludes us. We end up in a cycle of endless pursuit, never truly satisfied, leading to mental health struggles.

Modern life is full of what psychologists call the Progress Paradox. Despite technological advancements, improved living standards, and countless conveniences, people are less happy and sicker than they were decades ago. In fact, studies show that levels of anxiety, depression, and dissatisfaction are on the rise. The reason for this paradox is simple: as we achieve more externally, we expect those achievements to lead to happiness. But external success only provides temporary pleasure, which is fleeting (hedonic). We then set our sights on the next goal, creating a never-ending cycle of doing without ever truly being.

Dr. Goswami says in his books that our thoughts and feelings, which he calls "quantum consciousness," can help shape what happens in our lives. We can then move away from the pursuit of external pleasure and instead focus on cultivating an inner state of peace and contentment.

Quantum science offers us a way out of this paradox.

WHAT IS TRUE HAPPINESS?

True happiness, as both quantum science and spiritual traditions like Buddhism suggest, comes from a state of *being*, not *doing*. This means that by changing how you are *being*, you can act differently and *do* things in another way, that actually allows you to *have* different results or things. It's the "Be, Do, Have" model (an unpredictable, full-of possibilities model, like quantum physics).

Remember, **we're human BEINGs, not human DOINGs.** It says it right there!

As the Buddha once said, "The greatest suffering comes from the ignorance of the true nature of reality." This ignorance, this misunderstanding of reality, leads us to focus on external things, achievements, and fleeting pleasures rather than seeking inner peace and lasting fulfillment.

The "Be, Do, Have" model allows us to think outside the box by focusing on our being. This gives us many possibilities of ways of "doing" things. And usually, these new actions make you act in the same frequencies as what you want.

As quantum physics shows, it's all about frequencies.

Just as mentioned in my story, the Quantum Entanglement research showed how things that are linked keep on changing in the same ways. The same frequencies work together, no matter the distance, influencing each other instantaneously.

BUT WHY DON'T WE ALREADY ACT THIS WAY?

You see, human doing is related to pleasure, which is temporary and dependent on external circumstances. It's the kind of happiness we get from buying a new car, receiving a promotion, or enjoying a delicious meal. These moments of pleasure are short-lived and often leave us wanting more.

On the other hand, being is about real inner happiness, the kind that comes from aligning with your true nature, feeling connected to the world around you, and finding peace in the present moment. This type of happiness is not dependent on external factors; it's a state of inner harmony and connection.

WHAT DOES IT MEAN TO FEEL CONNECTED?

Spirit isn't something mysterious or hard to reach—it's just how we feel in our soul. Imagine that warm feeling when you're with people you love or that peaceful sensation when you're watching a sunset or thinking about life's big questions. That's your soul feeling connected.

This connection can be to different things: a higher power, nature, or even a sense of purpose in the universe. People might call it spirituality, but it's really just a way of tuning in to something bigger than ourselves. When we do this, it helps us feel happier and stronger, inside and out.

WHY DOES FEELING CONNECTED MATTER?

Feeling connected is important because it reminds us of the idea that everything is One, a belief shared by many spiritual traditions. This concept is also echoed in quantum physics, which suggests that everything in the universe is linked in a web of connections. Imagine it like a giant spider web where every part is connected to every other part.

When we feel connected to nature, other people, and the world around us, studies show that we tend to be happier, live longer, and feel more satisfied with life. This sense of connection helps us reconnect with our spirit, which is what spirituality is all about. It's like feeling a warm hug from the universe, reminding us that we're never truly alone.

Recent research published in my first scientific paper shows a direct link between inner happiness and longevity. When we focus on our inner well-being, we not only improve our mental and emotional health but also enhance our physical health. This reinforces the idea that happiness is not just a fleeting emotion but a vital component of long-term health and vitality.

THE PRACTICAL TOOL: QUANTUM CONSCIOUS AWARENESS

Now that we've explored the difference between the classical and quantum views of reality, let's talk about how you can apply this shift to rethink your own life. The key to breaking free from the glass prison isn't just understanding quantum physics intellectually but experiencing it. This requires a fundamental shift in how we perceive the world and ourselves.

One powerful tool that can help facilitate this shift is the practice of conscious awareness. It's about bringing your attention to the present moment and recognizing that your thoughts, feelings, emotions, and perceptions are constantly shaping your reality. It's about becoming aware of the quantum field of possibilities and recognizing that you have the power to influence it.

Here's how you can start practicing conscious awareness today:

1. Remember Your Influence: Write a simple note on a Post-it to remind yourself that you have the power to change your world. Think of it like this: when you smile at someone, they often smile back. This is like the "quantum entanglement" and "observer effect" in science, showing that your actions and thoughts can affect what happens around you.

2. Pause and Reflect: Throughout your day, take moments to pause and reflect on your thoughts, feelings, and emotions. Are you operating from a place of fear, scarcity, or separation? Or are you aligned with the understanding that you are part of an interconnected, quantum reality where infinite possibilities exist?

3. Visualize the Quantum Field: Spend a few minutes each day imagining yourself as part of a big energy field, like being part of a giant web that connects everything. Picture energy flowing through you and out into the world, touching everything you meet. This helps you feel connected and see life as full of endless possibilities. (I've prepared an audio that can be easily followed).

4. Embrace Uncertainty: Understand that not knowing everything is okay. Understand that the universe is full of surprises. In fact, it's exciting! Instead of being scared of not knowing what's next, think of it as an exciting adventure. Imagine uncertainty as a door to new adventures. When you stop trying to control everything, you open yourself to amazing possibilities and changes. Picture yourself standing at a door, ready to step into a world of endless opportunities!

By practicing conscious awareness, you begin to rewire your perception of reality; you become a new observer. You'll start to see the world not as a fixed, material place but as a fluid, interconnected field of energy and possibility. This shift in perception is the key to breaking free from the glass prison. It's about realizing that the boundaries we've placed on ourselves are constructs of a materialistic, Newtonian worldview. The shift to quantum thinking allows us to see ourselves as part of an interconnected, energetic universe where everything is possible.

CONCLUSION: BREAKING FREE FROM THE GLASS PRISON FOR YOURSELF AND THE NEXT GENERATION

As we've explored, the glass prison is the invisible trap many of us live in a life driven by doing instead of being. It's the constant pursuit of happiness through external achievements rooted in a limited, outdated understanding of reality. The solution, as quantum science and spiritual wisdom teach us, is not to *do* more but to *be* more. To shift from a mindset of doing to a state of being, where we align with our true nature and understand the interconnectedness of everything.

But this journey is not just for us as adults; it's one we must embark on with our children. As parents, teachers, mentors, or caregivers, we have a responsibility to model and teach the next generation foundational skills that will allow them to navigate life from a place of inner happiness, resilience, and balance. This wisdom is timeless and can set our kids on a healthier trajectory.

Children, like us, are growing up in a world that often values "doing" over "being." As adults, we must teach them that true happiness isn't found in constant striving or external success but in understanding the power of their own consciousness. Helping kids cultivate conscious awareness and understand their connection to the world around them will give them lifelong tools for emotional health and resilience.

The lessons we teach our kids now will shape their health, both mentally and physically, for the rest of their lives. By shifting away from the traditional, materialistic mindset and embracing quantum principles of consciousness and being, we're not only breaking free from our own glass prisons but ensuring the next generation grows up with the tools to create a healthier, happier, and more balanced life.

This is the ultimate solution to happiness: not just for ourselves but for our children, families, and society as a whole. Let's start breaking down those glass walls and help our kids grow in a world where they can thrive, connected to their true potential and healthy for life.

If you're ready to dive deeper into these concepts, I invite you to join me on my book resource page, where you will find some deeper explanations and guided exercises. Let's continue this journey together, learning the wisdom and skills that will not only transform our lives but also the lives of the children we love. Sign up here: https://www.vitaquantum.com/healthyforkids

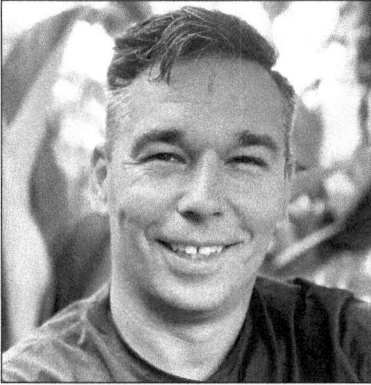

Philippe Brouillard is an expert in quantum happiness, quantum manifestation, and quantum health, offering transformative online programs that guide individuals toward inner fulfillment by blending science and spirituality. He is the author of the book « Rethinking Life » (When Quantum Science and Spirituality Join: Happiness Materializes).

From a young age, Philippe was a visionary, questioning the status quo and seeking the deeper meaning of life. Labeled as gifted in school, he felt disconnected and bored, which pushed him into the adrenaline of extreme sports, where he ranked #21 in mogul skiing in Canada. But then, even as he built a thriving conscious health business with his father, Dr. Brouillard, and his wife, Natasha Azrak IFMCP, Philippe felt that something was missing.

His lifelong quest for answers led him to study NLP, Hypnotism, Integral Life Coaching, Shamanism, etc., but it was the discovery of Quantum Science that provided the key to integrating science and spirituality. Inspired by the Dalai Lama's words, "Spirituality without Quantum physics is an incomplete picture of reality," Philippe closed his successful seven-figure business to pursue full-time a PhD in Quantum Science of Health, Prosperity, and Happiness.

Now, Philippe empowers others to transcend limiting beliefs and tap into their subconscious potential. His mission is to guide individuals toward living their best lives by connecting science and spirituality for true transformation and happiness.

He is also passionate about creating a Quantum EcoVillage, where it's second nature to be healthy because of surroundings allowing human evolution and nature to come together in harmony.

As an international speaker in both French and English, Philippe is known for simplifying complex concepts, helping others understand and apply quantum principles in their lives with ease. His teachings inspire lasting change and happiness on both personal and global levels.

Connect with Philippe: https://www.vitaquantum.com/link

CHAPTER 19

SENSORY SYMPHONY

ADOPTING SOUND PRACTICES FOR EMOTIONAL BALANCE

Francesca MacDonald, iah.fit co-founder

MY STORY

I'll never forget her tired face, masked with fear and confusion. Isla was a presence I felt destined to nurture since birth, a journey no book could have prepared me for.

Welcoming Isla into our family was a leap into the unknown, redefining our understanding of love and resilience. "Mommy, today is finally here! The day we've dreamed of for so long." My son's excited voice echoed our four-year anticipation. His small, moist hand clutched mine tightly as we walked briskly through the crisp morning air, each step closer to our long-held vision. *More than half his age has been spent picturing this little girl,* I mused, as my heart swelled with hope for the soul we were about to embrace.

Tears welled as I recalled our first glimpse of Isla in Haiti two years earlier. My husband, Michael, and I saw her briefly among thirty other children, each yearning for affection and a morsel to ease their hunger. The room buzzed with flies, and stray dogs wandered in and out, painting a stark picture of her world. My legs trembled, palms slick with sweat. *I wish the boys were here,* I thought, as this timid little girl was brought to our meeting place in the crèche. Outside, armed guards stood watch while a tropical sunset painted the sky—a fitting backdrop for this anticipated moment.

Fast-forward to October 8, 2024. The house was invitingly quiet. Michael sat across from me, our laptops primed for juicy work. "Here's your coffee, amore," I told him, my spirit alight with enthusiasm. Writing has always been my creative outlet. As the meeting with our publisher began, anticipation tingled through me. "Write a message to someone you love dearly," she instructed, urging simplicity and honesty. At that moment, as if guided by an unseen hand, Isla's name surfaced in my heart, and I found myself prepared to embrace the words I longed to share. The familiar scent of freshly brewed coffee stirred my emotions, directing my fingers to the keyboard.

Dear Isla (a pseudonym),

I want you to know that although things didn't go as planned, they unfolded as they were meant to. I dreamt of our first meeting and the wonders I longed to share with you—things to teach, sights to show, and adventures to embark on together. I was determined to create a life filled with balance and joy for you so the hardships of your early years would fade into distant memories. I wished to transform your tears into precious gems, treasures in your memory chest.

I imagined gently washing away the frightening images you saw, clearing your ears of unsettling sounds, your lungs of the thick dust you inhaled, and your system of the contaminated water you consumed. I pictured making you laugh until you couldn't anymore, filling your tummy with nutritious food, and ensuring your limbs were sustained by more than mud pies. I often wondered about the day they found you, imagining the exact place and how you got there. Did someone bring you? Did you wander off, and is someone still looking for you? I wondered if your mom survived your delivery and got to hold you at least once. It pained me to see you didn't know how to touch another or even blow a kiss.

Do you remember when you used to grab our ears and squeeze them as hard as you could? Our ears would turn red and blue, but we cherished it because that was your special way of showing us love. You were never comfortable with loud noises, and one day, when a car backfired on our way to therapy, you screamed as if caught in a nightmare. Mommy stopped the car and gently approached you in the back seat. Do you remember how we both started taking deep, calming breaths together? Then we took silly breaths and eventually put on some fun music. Before long, we were both singing along!

Your little hands were insatiably curious, eager to touch everything. Yet, there were moments when the world seemed too overwhelming, like when our dog barked, or the lawn mower roared; your eyes would clamp shut, leaving you silent and unreachable. Watching you explore the world, I realized your need to smell everything turned the unfamiliar into the familiar.

My dear one, I adore you. You've revealed a love I never knew existed, and your resilience inspires me daily.

As I reached for a tissue, the meeting continued, yet my mind drifted into a vivid reverie. *I am not sure if I'll ever return to the conversation's flow,* I admitted to myself. Scenes flashed like fireworks on a warm Fourth of July night. I recalled playing the Little Red Riding Hood game, solving the animal's puzzle, and the boys laughing as my heart constricted each time we played the 'colors' game. I'd say, 'Look, Isla, this is yellow,' drawing a yellow line, and then, 'This is red,' drawing a red line. Her proud response was always 'red!' even when pointing to yellow. My mind agonized over her struggle to see things correctly. *What else didn't she perceive right?* Countless sleepless nights were spent thinking of those beautiful brown eyes, as deep as the ocean, burying stories no sane adult could recount without feeling a profound ache; eyes that projected scenes of Haiti's street life—filthy and frenzied. Those scenes fueled my yearning to connect with the children who still navigate those precarious roads, their lives as vulnerable as dry leaves on a thin tree branch at the end of autumn.

Like untuned instruments, Isla's senses often struggled to harmonize, creating dissonance between what she perceived and how she processed the world. In heightened states, she seemed adrift, unable to hear the music within, disconnected from reality. Yet, in moments of clarity, her internal orchestra found its rhythm, allowing her to connect with the world. We embraced her journey gracefully, cherishing the beauty and complexity of her unique challenges.

As the meeting concluded, I reflected on Isla's transformative influence, a catalyst for deep insight. Her presence substantially reshaped our understanding of love and resilience, imparting invaluable teachings. This revelatory experience has led me to explore sensory integration, unveiling new layers of compassion and discernment. It wasn't just about choosing whom to write to; it was an epiphany about her invaluable lessons, particularly in grasping emotional regulation and its significance for quality of life.

Love, as Lao Tsu wisely noted, "is of all passions the strongest, for it attacks simultaneously the head, the heart, and the senses." This love became the foundation of our journey, compelling me to equip her and the boys with the tools to thrive. While Haiti's environment was fraught with sensory overload, our modern society presents unique pressures that challenge emotional equilibrium. My gift to them would be the ability to find equanimity within themselves, recognize their optimal state, and identify potential disruptions to their well-being as they grow and expand their horizons. Love, resilience, and sensory experiences wove through our journey, redefining our family.

Later, I turned to my husband and exclaimed, "I just realized what I want for our children, amore!" He looked at me, surprised yet supportive. As a music producer, he appreciated my metaphor: "I envision our children navigating life as integral parts of a grand sensory symphony, harmonizing with the world within and around them," I declared.

Through our emotional challenges, we learned firsthand that when one's inner melody is not in sync, life becomes less enjoyable, moods fluctuate, and resilience weakens. I'm honored to share the tools we use in our family to try to be fine-tuned instruments. While it requires occasional reminders, we've found these skills invaluable for reducing anxiety during hyperactive states, preventing escalation, and serving as a rescue method when overwhelmed.

These insights are drawn from various resources, including countless books, research, videos, podcasts, and interactions with counselors and therapists. This work reflects my unique interpretation and perspective, shaped by life experiences and a broad exploration of brain biology, neurological workings, and psychological and holistic approaches. I hope these tools empower many; even helping a few would bring me immense joy.

THE SKILL

As I transition from sharing our profoundly personal journey with Isla to imparting a transformative skill, I invite you to become the maestro of your sensory symphony. Our senses are the portals through which we experience the world, and mastering them can significantly enhance our quality of life. From the earliest whispers of life in the womb, our sensory journey begins, laying the foundation for emotional and cognitive development. As we navigate the complexities of modern life, creating a harmonious sensory environment becomes essential for thriving.

During adolescence, the brain undergoes significant changes that shape our perception and interaction with the world. This period of heightened adaptability, known as neuroplasticity, allows the brain to form new connections and learn rapidly. However, it also makes teens more susceptible to impulsive behaviors and intense emotions. Understanding our senses' central role during this time allows us to develop strategies to maintain composure and support well-being.

Sound is paramount for self-regulation. Entrainment, the process of synchronizing biological rhythms with sound, helps align brainwaves, enhancing focus and reducing tension. In one of my favorite books, *Healing at the Speed of Sound*, authors Alex Doman and Don Campbell highlight sound's power, demonstrating how calming music can lower the stress hormone cortisol and alleviate anxiety.

In our family, humming or playing a favorite tune restores emotional balance. My boys naturally select ambient beats or instrumentals to focus on during tasks. Sound pollution heightens tension, so being mindful of our auditory environment is imperative. Michael thoughtfully fills our home with melodies that align with our moods and needs.

How often have you heard Thomas Jefferson's quote, 'Knowledge is power'? Rooted in the Latin 'advertere,' meaning 'to turn toward,' awareness goes beyond mere observation. It involves recognizing and understanding our thoughts, emotions, and surroundings, enhancing emotional stewardship, and allowing us to respond thoughtfully rather than impulsively. The **S.O.U.N.D.** acronym, a tool I created, seamlessly integrates into daily life. Initially designed to guide my children through adolescence, it now empowers Michael, me, and anyone who embraces it. This tool is invaluable when we feel sensory or emotional dysregulation setting in, helping us reverse potential overwhelm through effective strategies readily available within ourselves. All we need is the awareness to recognize and use them.

S.O.U.N.D.

S: Slow breathing manages overwhelming emotions. Breathing is unique because it can be both automatic and consciously controlled, allowing us to activate the parasympathetic nervous system (PNS) responsible for settling the body. Slow breathing engages lung stretch receptors, sending soothing signals through the vagus nerve—a vital nerve that connects the brain to the body, influencing heart rate and digestion. This process reduces heart rate and promotes relaxation. Imagine using slow breathing before a test or presentation to notice its calming effect.

Quick Action Reminder: Deep inhale, slow exhale.

O: Observing patterns: When we aim to change a pattern, the process involves neuroplasticity, where the brain forms new connections and pathways. By consciously identifying stress triggers, we can disrupt old patterns and create new, healthier ones. For example, when feeling anxious about a blood test, focusing on the positive aspect of enjoying breakfast afterward can help shift the emotional response. This practice gradually rewires the brain, making it easier to adopt beneficial patterns over time.

Quick Action Reminder: Spot patterns; create more soothing ones.

U: Use Humming: Humming creates chest vibrations that stimulate the vagus nerve, enhance vagal tone, and influence heart rate, digestion, and relaxation. Humming also increases nitric oxide production, improving blood flow and reducing blood pressure. By extending the exhalation phase naturally, humming encourages mindfulness and reduces stress-related thoughts. During a stressful doctor's visit, I hum softly to calm my nerves and focus on breathing, finding immediate relief.

Quick Action Reminder: Hum softly to relax.

N: Naming emotions, known as affect labeling, aids self-regulation by calming the amygdala, the brain's emotional center, reducing the intensity of emotional responses. Verbalizing feelings creates a sense of distance from the emotion, allowing for a more thoughtful response rather than a reactive one. Regularly naming emotions reinforces neural pathways that support emotional management, making it easier to handle them effectively. When overwhelmed, I say, "I'm feeling anxious," which helps me acknowledge the emotion and take steps to manage it.

Quick Action Reminder: Label feelings to reduce intensity.

D: Dopamine, a crucial neurotransmitter in the brain's reward system, is essential for pleasure and mood regulation. Maintaining balanced dopamine levels helps manage stress and emotional triggers. Physical movement, positive visualization, and music boost dopamine, enhancing mood and reducing stress. Simple exercises like walking, stretching, listening to mid-frequency, calming music, or even anticipating the musical climax of a favorite song can stimulate dopamine release, fostering a cycle of pleasure and satisfaction. My daily workouts are my go-to for a healthy dopamine boost.

Quick Action Reminder: Move, visualize, and enjoy music.

The S.O.U.N.D. acronym we just learned is an indispensable rescue tool. It helps us manage emotional escalation when triggers arise. It provides immediate support, allowing us to regain control in challenging situations.

Let's transition to the core knowledge of the **6 L's for Learning**. Imagine equipping young adults with a toolkit akin to a Boy Scout's essentials for the wilderness. As a scout wouldn't venture into the wild without a pocket knife and compass, we shouldn't navigate life without these foundational skills. The *6 L's* offer a deeper understanding of what triggers our system and how to manage it, empowering us to master our emotional regulation. By mastering the *6 L's*, we reduce our reliance on the S.O.U.N.D. technique, fostering a more resilient self, ready to face life's challenges with composure and grace.

LEARN YOUR TRIGGERS

Understanding what stresses you is critical to managing emotions. Triggers are situations that spark stress responses, like increased cortisol and adrenaline. You can use your brain's adaptability to create calming pathways by identifying triggers. This awareness helps you anticipate stress, make proactive choices, and build fortitude. For example, if a deadline causes anxiety, plan tasks ahead to turn stress into manageable steps.

Quick Glance Reminder: Identify stressors and plan ahead.

LEARN YOUR TOLERANCE

Understanding your stress tolerance is imperative to maintaining emotional poise. Everyone has different thresholds for stimuli like noise and stimulants, which, when exceeded, can disrupt well-being. For example, if sound is a stressor for you, taking "sound breaks" with calming natural sounds can help restore peace. You can develop strategies like noise-canceling headphones or managing screen time to prevent stress escalation and maintain balance by identifying your unique tolerance levels.

Quick Glance Reminder: Know your limits with stimuli.

LEARN SELF-REINFORCEMENT

Understanding and responding to your body's internal signals, known as interoception, is fundamental to self-awareness and emotional steadiness. By tuning into cues like hunger, thirst, or fatigue, you strengthen neural pathways that enhance your ability to meet your body's needs. This practice aids self-regulation and reinforces a sense of self-worth, signaling to your brain and body that you are attentive and caring. For example, if you notice tension building in your shoulders, taking a moment to stretch and breathe acknowledges your body's signals, promoting relaxation and reinforcing your brain's sense of control and your body's trust in your care.

Quick Glance Reminder: Listen to your body's cues.

LEARN YOUR MEMORIES

Memories, especially emotional ones, shape mood and behavior. You can manage your emotional responses more effectively by identifying sensory triggers linked to these events. For instance, a loud noise might evoke a stressful memory, causing anxiety. Neuroplasticity allows you to modify memories and form new associations. Forgetting isn't about erasing memories but involves relearning. Engaging different senses in this process can help create new associations, like associating a scent with a happy memory, which can uplift your mood during challenging times.

Quick Glance Reminder: Recognize memory cues; form new links.

LEARN YOUR BRAIN

Understanding brain development empowers you to regulate emotions by identifying which brain part is active in various situations. The *reptilian brain* governs survival instincts, often triggering fight-or-flight responses. The *rat brain* handles emotions and memories, leading to impulsive reactions. The *monkey brain* is responsible for reasoning and problem-solving, enabling thoughtful responses. By recognizing which part is in charge, you can consciously shift control to your monkey brain, steering your emotions rather than being driven by them. My young son once said, "Sorry, Mommy, I wasn't using my monkey brain," acknowledging his impulsive reaction. Recognizing when your monkey brain is overwhelmed allows you to reengage it effectively.

Quick Glance Reminder: Engage your brain with mindfulness.

LEARN YOUR STRONGEST SENSE

Understanding your strongest sense helps tailor stress management. We all have sensory preferences, naturally relying more on one sense to perceive and interact with the world. To identify your dominant sense, notice which sensory input you rely on most when learning or calming yourself—do you prefer seeing, hearing, or touching? You can create personalized coping mechanisms and learning strategies by focusing on your dominant sense. For example, if you have a visual preference, you might use visual aids to manage stress. In contrast, if you have a strong sense of smell, use essential oils to create a calming environment.

Quick Glance Reminder: Utilize your dominant sense for regulation.

"When you understand that nothing is missing, the entire world is yours." – Lao Tzu. This profound quote encapsulates the essence of achieving balance through sensory awareness. By nurturing your senses, you can orchestrate a sensory symphony that reveals life's fullness, realizing everything you need is already within you.

Integrate the S.O.U.N.D. and *6 L's for Learning* frameworks into your daily routine. Begin with one technique, practice it consistently, and witness the transformation in your emotional mastery and personal growth. Share these insights with loved ones, empowering them to navigate life's complexities with confidence and self-reliance. Remember, the journey to a balanced and fulfilling life starts with a single step—take that step today and unlock your potential.

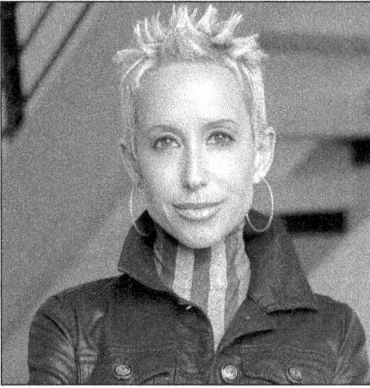

Francesca MacDonald is the visionary Co-Founder of iah.fit, a transformative platform dedicated to inspiring holistic well-being through frequency music, art, and heart-centered AI. As a passionate content creator and blog author for iah.fit, she shares insights to empower others.

With a background in personal development, Francesca previously owned Dynamic Personal Growth, a motivational venture. Born and raised in Venice, Italy, she studied Asian languages and is a polyglot with a Diploma in Sports Nutrition. Her life philosophy, "Why not?" drives her fearless pursuit of freedom and excellence, reminding everyone that limitations are self-imposed.

Francesca is passionate about crafting engaging narratives for children and teens. She also dedicates her talents to writing on wellness topics, inspiring readers of all ages. Her love for poetry reflects her profound appreciation for the written word and its transformative power.

Her philanthropic spirit shines through her efforts in facilitating the opening of a school in Haiti, providing education, meals, and shelter for children.

Francesca's vibrant personality is reflected in her love for fashion, daily workouts, and unique Italian flair—ironing everything but skipping pasta and pizza. She cherishes being her boys' best friend and biggest fan and dreams of experiencing all Cirque du Soleil shows. Married to her soulmate, Michael, for 23 years, Francesca's life revolves around making a meaningful impact.

Connect with Francesca:

Websites:

https://iah.fit/francesca-macdonald/

https://www.francescamacdonald.com/

Email:

Francesca@iah.fit

Facebook:

https://www.facebook.com/profile.php?id=61565455178381

Inspirations:

Brain Rules for Baby by John Medina

Brainstorm by Daniel J. Siegel M.D.

Healing at the Speed of Sound by Don Campbell and Alex Doman

CHAPTER 20

THE GIFT OF BODY AWARENESS

A WAY TO CLEAR TENSION AND FIND EASE IN YOUR BODY

Maryann Herklotz, PT, RCST

MY STORY

I'm seeking treatment from a new practitioner to help me with odd new symptoms. Sitting in his treatment room for a mere five minutes, he asks, "Can I place my hand here?" Pointing to my sternum, he says, "There's something there." I say, "Sure," yet I have no clue what he's talking about. He places three finger pads on the center of my chest and casually instructs, "Okay, cry."

Before the complete sentence comes out, "What do you mean by. . ." I'm sobbing. Everything disappears around me, and the saltiest tears I can remember fall straight down into the corners of my mouth. A half minute later, the tears stop. He says, "Nah, there's more." *Here I go again*. There *are* more. "Alright, moving on," he says as he proceeds to check the alignment of my neck.

Seriously. What just happened?

That is not, I'll repeat, **not** how I practice.

I'm about to teach you what I understand about body awareness and humbly share that I was once quite unaware of my body. That moment, sixteen years ago, I directly experienced how our bodies have the capacity to hold more than purely physical impact and tension. They hold stories, emotions, and experiences that may serve a purpose of protection at the time. But when they're no longer helpful, we can release them.

By the way, the unusual symptoms (headaches, tingling, fatigue, and vertigo) I sought treatment for turned out to be caused by a tick-borne infection. That session with a practitioner who I was told by a trusted friend, "You have to see him, he'll help," did help. He didn't diagnose the ehrlichiosis, but he did help me release something—immediately making me feel a little lighter. Those tears, even if unrelated to the tick infection, created a heaviness I hadn't been aware of until they were released. Those tears, and whatever may have been behind them, needed to come out.

OPENING A DOOR

I recall the moment I first heard about visceral manipulation. It opened a new path in my life. This was in 2008. I was sitting in the staff room of the cancer hospital where I was working when my colleague approached me and said, "Mar, do you want to take this class with me?" as she handed me a trifold pamphlet. It described a form of manual therapy that addressed the interconnection of our organs to all other structures in our body through fascia (connective tissue), nerves, vessels, ligaments, muscles, etc. I'm fascinated. I'm introduced to motility, a natural and continuous movement of a healthy (in this case) organ toward and away from the center of our bodies in a rhythmic harmony with other organs. Whenever movement is restricted in an area, the local imbalance can cause a disruption elsewhere in our bodies. "Sign me up." We took that first class together.

Learning about visceral manipulation was what first exposed me to "listening" to the body through its tissues. Listening means placing a hand on the body to feel a pull toward the area of greatest tension, where there is a lack of movement, which may be causing an impact on overall well-being. That site may be an organ, nerve, bone, ligament, or within the central nervous system, and there may be a connection between two or more areas. As the developer of this work, Jean Pierre Barral, DO, MRO(F), RPT, describes, the client has their story (of what they are feeling, when their concern started, etc.). However, the body knows the story. "Only the tissues know."

Listening to what my hands feel soon became primary in my manual therapy assessments. My thinking mind expecting something may not be as accurate. In every case, I want to hear my client's concerns, learn their history, and then listen with my hands to allow the body to share its story. For example, a patient has pain in her neck, and I'm directed via listening to her lower back. The first area I will contact is her lower back, even if she has no story related to that area. Why? The body is picking up an area of tension that may correspond with the neck pain. As practitioners, we must listen and follow, through our hands, to where the body is guiding us.

Here is an example: I went for a treatment session soon after my first class for injuries from distance running. I had right knee and right foot pain. Still limited in my body awareness, I had just finished running 18 miles with a stress fracture in my right foot while doing a long run in preparation for a marathon. I felt a *little ache* at the time.

During this session, I learned that a restriction in my diaphragm created a line of tension down through my right side, causing a misalignment of my knee and foot. Releasing the restriction in my diaphragm improved my alignment. My stress fracture needed time to heal, but since then, running hasn't caused pain in either area again. That was it! My gastroesophageal reflux disappeared, too, but that felt like a bonus.

Incorporating this treatment approach into my patient care was powerful. My patients' long-term aches, pains, and conditions in their musculoskeletal, gastrointestinal, lymphatic, and nervous systems improved right away.

Listen and follow. Trust where I am guided. Got it. I'm hooked.

The contact is gentle, even subtle, but very precise. I needed to deepen my study of anatomy and my ability to connect with and sense the anatomy under my hands.

I took class after class and studied other paths, including craniosacral therapy, nerve and vascular manipulation, and biodynamic craniosacral therapy. These are all forms of osteopathy. The body is viewed as a whole, and the diagnosis and treatment are carried out by the hands. Finding the root cause of symptoms and treating it restores health and balance wherever possible.

I continued working in the hospital for thirteen years after beginning this training. I took up to six seminars each year, each full of rich material. I received countless manual therapy sessions because experiencing the work helped me better understand it. As a supervisor, I did less patient care in the hospital, so I began seeing clients after work to stay connected with this training. My vision of opening a private practice was starting to clarify. I was appreciative of my role in the hospital. I felt blessed, but I had also begun to feel stifled. It felt like I was growing out of my clothes and shoes yet still trying to fit into them.

OUR BODIES ARE METAPHORS. WHAT IF WE ASK WHAT THEY'RE TRYING TO TELL US?

In early 2021, I received a craniosacral session from a practitioner who knew me well. My body directed her to my diaphragm and the muscles of my ribcage. She said, "It feels like you are not taking full breaths." It was true; my breath was unusually shallow. I said, "It feels like I'm wearing a corset tied tightly around my ribs." While I don't recall when this sensation began, I do know that I felt restricted and limited in my current role. The restricted breath seemed to mirror my sense that I couldn't expand at work.

I left the hospital in December 2021 to open my private practice. On the last day of my 20-year tenure, I felt immense gratitude and joy. I was proud of my accomplishments and elated for what would be. Two blocks away from the hospital, heading toward the subway to go home one final time from that role, my eyes widened with recognition. I gasped with awe. Something changed in me, rather, on me—*the corset is gone!* I never looked back.

It seems to me that once the therapist oriented me to the restriction she identified in my diaphragm and released it physically, it freed me up in some way. Perhaps this supported my decision to move forward when I did.

As a practitioner, I've experienced many similar situations. Here's an example. My client described a pain in her shoulder that felt stabbing in quality as if a knife had been placed there. About halfway into the session, as my hands were on her shoulder, it felt like something came up and tapped the palm of one of my hands. Next, I felt a warmth, and the tissues around her shoulder softened. We made eye contact, and she said, "The knife is out." I acknowledged, "Yes, I believe so." She left without pain.

Three months after that session, she called to share that she had let go of anger, grief, and the physical pain that she felt for a long time. She also wanted me to know about a big move she made in her life that she'd wanted to make but hadn't felt ready until recently.

ORIENTING TO THE HEALTH

A few months after leaving the hospital, I'm sitting in a biodynamic craniosacral class with my teachers and colleagues, sharing how nourishing the work can be. The teacher said four words that brought me so much peace and a sense of being where I belonged at that moment. She said, in this work, "We hold the health." I couldn't hear anything else for the next few minutes. My eyes welled up. *We hold the health. I spent twenty years in a hospital environment holding the disease. Now I am holding the health. I am exactly where I need to be. Thank you.*

Biodynamic craniosacral therapy brought my awareness deeper and added to the way I can approach my treatment sessions. This work focuses on tuning into another expression of health, the subtler tide-like rhythm felt throughout the body from the movement of fluid deep within the central nervous system as it is expressed through the tissues. Sensing this rhythm and any disruption of it can point to where there may be imbalances, tension, or fulcrums in the body. When I incorporate this work, I'm even lighter in my touch, listening, and allowing. I give the tissues space and allow healing to unfold.

RETURNING TO THE HEART

"If words come out of the heart, they will enter the heart."

~ Rumi

In 2023, while receiving a session in class, my colleague was drawn to work near my sternum. *Here we are again.* However, now fifteen years after that first experience, this was different. I felt a line of tension and a burning sensation that accompanied it. *Is it my phrenic nerve?* I often want to name the anatomy when I receive a session. It started from underneath my collarbone, down the front of my chest, to beneath the ribs on my left side, just over my heart. The tension continued to build. It was pretty intense this time until finally, after several minutes, it released. My body relaxed as everything softened. It felt like my heart expanded and took up more space. My organs around it moved over, saying, "Make room; here she comes!" I said to myself, *I don't have to hold that anymore.*

The chicken or the egg, what came first? Was the cause emotional or an old physical strain that affected the path of the nerve? I don't know, but I do know something old let go and I felt an incredible sense of freedom and relief. The cause is not always clear. What matters is the tissues know.

I work with plenty of clients who come in for purely structural concerns. When the structural tensions are released, the treatment feels complete, and their symptoms fully resolve. However, through this work, we may recognize non-physical tensions that are also being held in the body. While we do not look for them, these will show up and release only when the client is open and ready. I always meet each client where they are at that moment.

I now feel this work is all about the heart. This work has opened mine in more ways than I can describe. When we free ourselves of holding these extra tensions in our bodies, it feels to me that we can get closer to our hearts.

THE SKILL

WHAT DOES IT MEAN TO BE BODY-AWARE?

To be body-aware means that I am sensing what I feel in the present moment. I'm aware of what is happening in real time.

Here are two examples:

It can mean: I feel calm. I have a sense of harmony in my body. I feel my feet on the ground. My breath is slow and relaxed. My thoughts are clear. I'm aware of my environment, for example, the temperature, smells, and sounds. I'm patient with and available to those in my company. Overall, I feel a sense of ease.

Or it can mean: I'm about to go into a job interview. *I am nervous.* My throat feels tight. My voice is shaky. My breath is shallow. My palms are sweating. I'm fully prepared, but my body perceives something here as a threat.

Being body-aware allows us an opportunity to be in control of our circumstances. As in the second example, I can acknowledge the nervousness that arises and take a moment to settle and resource myself, which may lead to a better outcome in the interview.

WHAT MY WORK HAS TAUGHT ME ABOUT BODY AWARENESS

I need to be aware of my state of presence before I work with a client. I focus on being heart-centered and anchored. This allows me to be present with them yet spacious, meaning having no agenda or expectation. What arises is meant to arise. Creating a safe, nurturing space for my client allows for the fullest potential of healing in that session. And, if my client begins to process a challenging emotion or experience, the more grounded and centered I become, the more supported they will feel in the process.

Because of something called neuroception, our nervous systems are constantly working behind the scenes to pick up cues from our environment and social interactions to answer a question. That question is, "Am I safe?" It's important to note that our perceptions of threat vs. safety may differ based on our histories and experiences. In short, our nervous systems are constantly checking in with each other. This happens in all relational situations.

In a relationship, for example, a parent and child, when safety is felt, co-regulation can occur. Broadly described, co-regulation is when two people together create an environment that supports the emotional well-being of one another.

THE GIFT

I should now tell you what the "gift" of body awareness is, as my title implies. The gift is when we are present with what we are feeling, and in a friendly-observant way, we allow it an opportunity to change. Something heavy may lighten or tight may become more open and spacious. Just as I observe time and again in my work, we heal because we face what we are ready to heal, and we can also do this for ourselves.

WHY AM I TEACHING YOU ABOUT BODY AWARENESS?

I believe that when we are body-aware, we can better support ourselves. In turn, we become more available and supportive of others, such as those children and loved ones in our world, as our nervous systems meet with one another.

I encourage the understanding that we will sometimes lose this sense of awareness. There is no perfection, and nothing is constant. We can choose to hold ourselves and others with compassion, knowing that when we give ourselves space and practice again, we can return to being more aware.

FINDING YOUR ANCHOR

To me, an anchor symbolizes stability, peace, and safety. It reminds me that a sense of home is always available to me. This resources me and, in return, helps me to be a better resource for others. I hope this helps you as well.

- Start by finding a comfortable position to be in for a few moments.
- What is the general sense of your body at this moment? (For example, tired, heavy, light, relaxed, at ease)
- Imagine a line from the crown of your head, down your back, all the way to your feet. Does that feel supportive for you in this present moment? If so, maybe that becomes an anchor. Otherwise, perhaps you prefer to use the connection of your feet with the ground as your anchor. These are suggestions. Think of what feels suitable for you in terms of an anchor. Remember, this is simply something to keep you present in this moment.
- Once you find your anchor, be with it for a few breaths.
- Tune into your breath. Is there anything that you notice about your breath?
- Begin to widen your attention to your whole body, moving out from your anchor.

- Do you notice any particular area/sensation; what stands out? Is there a quality that feels important to know about? If so, can you name it? For example, tight shoulders. Naming what you notice can be helpful.

- Keep an awareness of your anchor while asking yourself if there is a possibility of softening (in this case, tight shoulders). Can you send breath into the area? Take as much time as you need.

- After a few rounds of breath, check in. Did anything change? What are the sensations and qualities now? What about the quality of your breath?

- Keep a friendly awareness. Notice what you are feeling without any judgment.

- You can repeat the last three steps as many times as you'd like.

- Eventually, return to your anchor and know it is accessible anytime you want a reminder of that support.

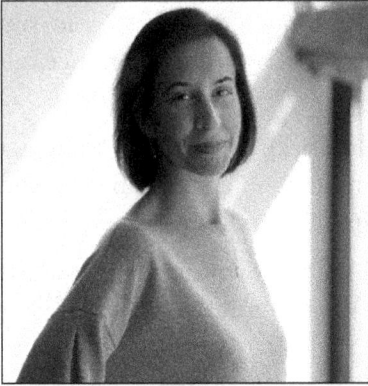

Maryann Herklotz, PT, RCST, is a native New Yorker. She worked as a physical therapist in the oncology setting for twenty years at Memorial Sloan Kettering. She opened her private practice in early 2022, currently in New York City, and has been enjoying maintaining her practice while also working weekly with her first teacher/mentor of visceral manipulation and craniosacral therapy at his practice. While she holds several certifications in her field, the most relevant to her current practice is her certification in Biodynamic Craniosacral Therapy. She works with clients of all ages, from infants to older adults, using an osteopathic manual therapy approach to support their healing and overall well-being. She sees clients for a wide variety of health concerns. When she is not in New York City, she is visiting friends/family or traveling, often far away, to study this work and enjoy an adventure. As a hobby, she studied wine for many years, and holds a wine certification. This sparked her love for combining travel with learning as she toured the wine regions of different countries to explore their local culture, history, food, and overall beauty. While she is currently rooted in the city, her heart settles the moment she steps foot into the softness of nature. She feels incredibly fortunate to have clients who are led to work with her to facilitate their wellness and healing. The relationships with and support of her friends, family, loved ones, teachers, and colleagues are a continuously renewing resource for her.

Connect with Maryann:

Website: www.whitepinephysicaltherapy.com

FITNESS AND MOVEMENT

---

*"A man's health can be judged
by which he takes two at a time – pills or stairs."*

~ Jim Rohn

FITNESS AND MOVEMENT: AN OVERVIEW

Fitness—is the goal: it's our overall state of health and physical capability.

Exercise—is how we get there: it's the specific activities aimed at improving or maintaining fitness.

This pillar seems to be the hardest for many to embrace for several reasons: Exercise takes work. Inertia doesn't usually take us there. It takes time away from our day. And it often takes effective motivation, which we can't consistently rely on it to be present. The good news is that if we focus first on taking action, motivation often follows!

The consensus among all our Fitness Pillar authors is—**movement first!**

Movement means all types of motions, from your basic daily activities like walking and bending to structured exercises like lifting weights, running, or doing yoga. It's the essence of fitness because it keeps the body functional and adaptable, enabling you to perform daily tasks and physical challenges more efficiently and with less risk of injury.

Moving keeps the blood flowing and helps keep your hormones in balance. It improves your mood and thousands of other things behind the scenes. So when sitting all day, you're at a huge disadvantage.

The Fitness Tree

Fitness never comes from one thing. All these components are key to having your best physical function in life—for the long term.

As you create and implement an exercise plan, think about how you're building all these components of fitness: alignment, strength, agility, and endurance.

Alignment—the optimal positioning of the body's joints, muscles, and bones to move efficiently and effectively while minimizing strain and risk of injury. This includes having a proper posture!

The *kinetic chain* is the principle that all parts of the body are interconnected, meaning that movement in one part affects the entire system. When the body is properly aligned, it prevents undue stress on any single area by ensuring that movements are balanced and coordinated.

Strength—the ability of your muscles to lift, pull, push, and stabilize heavy things, including your own body. The more developed your muscles are (muscle mass) the stronger and safer you are, especially as you get older. Muscle mass also correlates with bone strength and is a key marker for health and longevity. The more you add weight/resistance as you move, the stronger you become.

Strength also relies on flexibility- the more flexible you are (think-stretching, and how much motion your joints have), the greater the ability to safely develop your strength.

Agility—the ability to move quickly and easily, allowing for rapid changes in direction while maintaining balance and control. You train this with activities that include coordination, balance, and reaction time.

Endurance—the ability of the body to sustain prolonged physical activity or exertion. This comes from how efficiently your heart and lungs can supply oxygen and energy to your muscles and entire body. Both aerobic exercises (dancing, running, cycling) and anaerobic exercises (weightlifting, sprinting) train your cardiovascular and muscular endurance.

Just like a tree, true fitness is built from a strong foundation and grows in all directions. As you nurture your fitness, you cultivate your own tree, strengthening it over time to grow even stronger, more flexible, and capable.

CHAPTER 21

AN ALIGNED LIFE
BEGINS WITHIN

THE IMPACT OF POSTURE
ON BODY AND MIND

Caitilin Twain, Health Coach, Movement and Breathwork Instructor

MY STORY

Every morning, in the dim light of the study, I braced myself for what I came to call "my 20 minutes of torture." What began as an early morning meditation practice was actually a stress regulation and endurance test, and no matter how much I dreaded it, I knew it was the medicine I needed. The room was silent except for the soft creak of the floorboards as I moved, careful not to wake my baby or toddler. I did some gentle stretching to smooth my stiff body, then settled onto a bolster—the backs of my hips, ribs, shoulders, and head pressed against the wall—and prepared to sit still for 20 minutes. My back muscles burned from the effort of holding an upright posture, but I persisted.

The fight was always the same: my will to sit upright clashed with a body determined to fold in on itself. I was physically weak from fighting Lyme Disease for the better part of the previous decade. My body was curved inward, my shoulders slumping forward from years of breastfeeding and stooping down to meet my toddler's needs. In addition to the self-sacrifice of motherhood, my body reflected the erosion of my self-esteem, worn down by years spent in a marriage where my own needs were invisible. I felt small and diminished—physically and emotionally.

In these moments of stillness, I began to see the cycle I was stuck in—poor posture reinforcing physical discomfort, which fed into my low confidence. Then, day by day, something began to shift. I noticed I could sit a little longer without pain and could breathe a little deeper. My back and belly grew stronger, and as they did, so did I. It wasn't just my posture that was changing—something was realigning within me. Each time I straightened my spine, I felt more confident and capable. I was cultivating strength, grace, and resilience by sitting quietly with safe discomfort.

I literally and figuratively grew a backbone.

Four years later, I was divorced and joined a yoga teacher training. By then, I had become a new person—I confidently modeled the discipline of self-care born out of self-love for my children. I knew those early morning "torture sessions" had a profound effect, but it was during the yoga teacher training that I began to learn how much they gave me.

I learned how deeply our body's systems are interconnected and why my realignment healed me not just physically but emotionally.

Not only do misalignments often result in pain and injury, they also limit our ability to breathe properly. Shallow breathing keeps us stuck in fight-or-flight mode. Over time, this can lead to chronic tension, anxiety, and depression. Realigning the bones doesn't just relieve pain; it creates proper breath mechanics, which shifts the body into a parasympathetic nervous system state, the "rest and digest" mode, where healing and clear thinking occur.

By stacking my rib cage correctly over my pelvis, I could breathe fully. I became grounded, clearer, and more centered. The choices I made—from leaving my marriage to navigating the challenges of single parenthood—came from a place of strength rooted in my body's alignment.

I came to feel how movement was the medicine I needed to repair from Lyme Disease and heal the parts of me that chose a loveless marriage. I became powerful and graceful, one of those yogis who could put her toes on her head while in a handstand. It was my intention to teach sweaty, intense yoga classes to large groups.

But the universe had other plans for me.

Very soon after becoming a yoga teacher, students asked me to teach them privately. At first, I was frightened by the level of responsibility I felt teaching one-on-one. Then I began to see that each new student was my next teacher, and I welcomed the opportunity to dive deep and learn what I needed to help whatever was presented to me: a frozen shoulder, a torn hamstring, high blood pressure, anxiety, cancer, diverticulitis, arthritis, and on and on. I did advanced yoga teacher training with a focus on scoliosis and back care, became certified in prenatal yoga, and took countless workshops with esteemed teachers. But mostly, I dove into books and the internet, learning all I could to help the incredible people who entrusted me with their bodies.

THE PAIN YOU FEEL IS OFTEN NOT WHERE IT ORIGINATES

One of the most transformative books I read was *Anatomy Trains* by Tom Myers. I learned that our bodies are connected through a web of tissue called fascia. Think of it as an interwoven sweater that gives the entire body its form. Just like with a sweater, when one area is pulled tight, it will have a tugging effect on the rest of the body. This explains why the pain we feel is often not where the problem originates.

When I started to work with bodies on a fascial level, students began to call me a "witch" or a "body whisperer."

Take Pam, who came to me with persistent neck pain. For years, she got regular massage and chiropractic adjustments, but the relief was only temporary. Instead of focusing on her neck, where she felt the pain, I showed her that the fascia in the front of her body was tight from repeatedly rounding forward. I taught her the value of stretching her entire body, but focused on the center of her chest, across her upper arms through her hands. This gave her the space she needed to strengthen her back muscles and ultimately move her bones into correct alignment. Once that was done, she no longer had neck pain, and she was liberated from the hamster-wheel of treat-repeat.

The hundreds of bodies I've worked with have shown me what scientists have now confirmed—we're born with different fascial constitutions. Our bodies run the spectrum from always-stiff-as-a-plank to hyper-mobile. Each body type needs an approach to movement that's different from the other.

The rigid warrior type would do well to focus on becoming more bendy and less breakable, while the willowy type should focus on strengthening and securing the joints.

No matter what the fascial constitution, I found that gentle movement, especially in the morning, can ease us into better alignment. Just like it's important to brush our teeth in the morning, good physical hygiene requires that we lengthen the fascia and lubricate the joints to prime the body for the day. The students who add this to their hygiene routine make much faster progress than those who don't.

I hope you'll try it yourself! Instead of thinking of muscle stretching, think of gently stretching and lengthening your entire body sweater in all directions so that you feel you have more room to breathe and move. If you don't have time to spare, find ways to move while you're waiting for the water to boil or talking with your kids about after-school plans.

When I'm short on time, my morning movement might look like me interlacing my fingers, turning the heels of my hands away, and lifting my arms. I might bend side to side, then flex and round my spine. I'll definitely make circles with my hips, bend and straighten my knees, and point and flex my feet, all while making coffee and evening plans with my partner. Ideally, I have seven minutes to spare to give my body a more comprehensive treat, and if you'd like to follow along, you can find such a session on my book landing page: https://www.ctwain.com/healthyforlife

Whether you're following along or letting your body move you, keep these principles in mind:

- Let your movements be gentle and inquisitive. Listen to your body and move only to the point where you feel a "stuckness." From there, come out of the stretch and then re-enter for a deeper pass.

- Move in sync with your breath. Initiate each expansive movement with an inhale and each contractive movement with an exhale. Never move to the point that your breath is stuck or inaccessible.

- Lubricate your joints by moving them in all the directions they were designed to go. When you move your joints, they're literally lubricated by something called synovial fluid. I think of the Tin Man oiling himself when I do this.

UNDERSTAND YOUR PAIN SIGNALS

The key concepts to note are gentleness, inquisitiveness, breath-initiated, and body-led.

I once had a student who was so zealous in her quest for perfect alignment that she tore her rotator cuff between our sessions. She thought that physical pain was an inevitable part of the human experience, especially while exercising. This isn't entirely true. While it's true that avoiding all discomfort can prevent growth, knowing the difference between productive and destructive pain is essential for healthy movement. Pain is your body's way of telling you that something is wrong, and ignoring pain can lead to injury.

When moving, there are three pain signals you should never ignore:

1. Pain near a joint during stretching. If you feel pain or the bulk of the stretch in your joints rather than the muscles, adjust until you feel the sensation in the belly of your muscle. This will keep your joints safe and lengthen the muscles, which is the real aim.

2. You can no longer breathe easily. If you're holding your breath or can't breathe freely, you're out of your comfort zone. Back off to a point where your breath remains long and steady.

3. You feel a sharp or zapping pain. This is likely nerve pain and should be addressed immediately by adjusting your position.

Whether in a class, with a personal trainer, or practicing on your own, your body is your best teacher. Pay attention to its pain signals, adjust so you are in correct alignment, and you'll progress safely. Stretching might "hurt so good," the muscles may burn when getting stronger, and the pain of releasing trauma buried within our fabric is rarely pleasant, but these are the kinds of pain that do indeed bring gain. Most others should be avoided.

WHAT YOU DO THE OTHER 23 HOURS COUNTS

Another main reason some students progress more quickly than others is they're better at keeping their postural awareness throughout the day.

Spending just an hour stretching and strengthening won't undo the damage of poor posture over the next 23 hours. Even if we put in good work during an exercise session, progress will be painfully slow if we slump over our phones and computers, use inadequate pillows when sleeping, and drive without actually using our headrests. One of the first things I do with my students is run a posture audit. We look at the areas they spend the most time in and make them more supportive of their bodies. That way the work they do with me can be reinforced the rest of the day, and progress is accelerated.

"TECH NECK"

Given the remarkable emotional transformations I've seen result from good alignment, I'm deeply concerned by the rising "tech neck" phenomenon—especially its prevalence in children and teens.

Tech neck refers to the slouched, forward-hunched posture that results from long hours spent looking down at phones and computers. Each of our bodies will take on different compensatory patterns to manage tech neck, but all of these compensations reduce our ability to breathe well and can lead to being stuck in the sympathetic (or fight-flight) nervous system. Tech neck also forces the back and neck muscles to be constantly working, which can only result in chronic tension, pain, and ultimately the dreaded hunchback. This pattern makes us more prone to injuries, resulting in a less active lifestyle, which certainly means a lower quality of life.

I fear a world where even our future leaders are increasingly trapped in a cycle of poor posture, diminished self-confidence, and reliance on medications for both pain and mood disorders. But we have a solution— when we're physically aligned, we're confident, calm, and strong. Through movement, we can find alignment and physically prepare our children and ourselves for emotional resilience and active longevity in pain-free bodies.

THE SKILL

You certainly don't have to do my "20 minutes of torture" to build yourself into correct posture, though that—when combined with intelligent movement—can get you there. There are many ways to nurture your body into a shape that's optimal, including yoga, martial arts, lifting, HIIT, running, etc. Not all bodies are the same, and not all forms of exercise are appropriate for everyone. It's important to find at least a few kinds of movements that are suited to your body type and personality. But what is universally true is that correct posture is the foundation of any movement regimen. Without good posture, you're setting yourself up for injury. But when you maintain good alignment, you'll be able to do whatever you want long into old age.

In order to find and maintain beautiful alignment in yourself, you first have to know what correct posture is. Optimal alignment when standing is when our ears, shoulders, hips, knees, and ankles are stacked in a straight line. The bottom of the entire rib cage should be stacked directly over the pelvis, which means your bottom low ribs do not stick out. Then, your weight should be evenly distributed between your heels, your big toe mounds, and your little toe mounds.

Take the posture test to see whether you have optimal alignment

1. Stand with your back against a wall with your heels just far enough from the wall to accommodate your butt. Place your feet hip bone distance apart, toes pointing forward.

2. Rest your hips, rib cage, backs of the upper arms, and middle of the back of your head into the wall.

3. Now, slide a hand between your lower back and the wall. There should be enough room for your hand, not much more. To accomplish this, some of you may feel like you have to do a pelvic tilt. Others of you will also feel your abs fire up powerfully as your low front ribs move down and in. There should be a sense of expansiveness in the low back rib cage, *not* a swooping away from the wall. This may be hard, but it is the most important piece of this puzzle because it sets you up for optimal breath mechanics. The only way to receive the full benefits of the breath is to stack the base of your ribcage over the bowl of your pelvis.

If you're able to easily rest the middle of the back of your head against the wall while maintaining all of the other contact points, you can safely do whatever physical pursuits you'd like, provided you're conscious of keeping your beautiful alignment, especially if you're lifting heavy objects.

If you found it very hard to pass this posture test, the good news is that you may have found the source of what ails you. I've seen students heal tinnitus, headaches, every kind of joint and muscle pain, GI issues, anxiety and *so* much more just from finding excellent alignment in all they do. And just as thrilling to me, I've witnessed profound emotional shifts as well.

Feel for yourself the connection between your posture and your emotional state.

Right now, fold in on yourself. Let your shoulders and head round forward. Let your gaze drift downward. Take ten breaths. Feel where your breath goes, where it ends. Notice your emotional state. Then, do the opposite. Sit tall. Press your feet into the floor to help you lengthen your spine even more. Stack the bottom of your rib cage over your pelvis, then your head over your rib cage. Lift your gaze to look at the horizon ahead of you. Now, breathe ten long breaths and again feel where your breath goes and where it ends. Notice your emotional state.

Were you able to take longer, deeper breaths when sitting tall? Did you notice a lift in your emotional state? Can you feel why it's so important to model and teach your child healthy alignment?

By creating a strong postural foundation for yourself, you, too, can find freedom from pain and live in a way that is aligned from within.

One of my students said it best:

"With everything in its right place, with my body aligned, I no longer have tension and pain. I'm just able to be the best version of myself with friends, family, colleagues, and even strangers. I'm just better mentally, a better version of myself."

For exclusive content, including videos guiding you through several of these exercises, go to https://www.ctwain.com/healthyforlife. I look forward to guiding you on your healing journey!

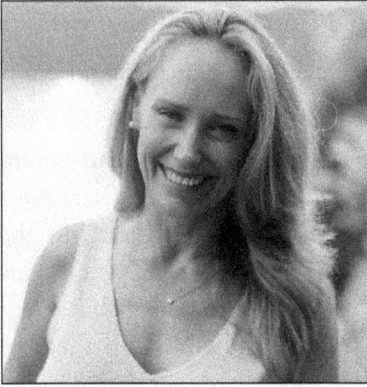

Caitilin Twain's unique teaching style is the result of her own battle with chronic Lyme Disease, a thyroid disorder, and 18 years of helping others heal. She's a certified Hatha and Prenatal Yoga Teacher. Her 300-hour advanced yoga studies focused on scoliosis and back care. Over the last 18 years, she's expanded her tool chest to include movement therapy, trigger point therapy, myofascial release, reiki, breathwork, and all things leading to microbiome health. She's certified to teach the Roll Model Method of self-myofascial release, is a graduate of the Institute of Holistic Integrative Studies Health Coaching Program, and is on her way to becoming a certified HeartMath Personal Resilience Mentor.

Based on years of study, healing herself as well as countless students, she developed the C. Twain Method, which blends modern science and ancient wisdom to help her students uncover the root causes of their pain and restore balance. She works with students across the globe who are facing health challenges and helps them tap into their inner resources to find complete healing. She encourages active participation from her students, and works in collaboration with their health team. Ultimately, her students become their own best healers.

Connect with Caitilin:

Website: https://www.ctwain.com

Instagram: https://www.instagram.com/caitilin_twain

Facebook: https://www.facebook.com/CTwainMethod

LinkedIn: https://www.linkedin.com/in/caitilin-twain-4b823721a/

YouTube: https://www.youtube.com/@Caitilin_Twain

CHAPTER 22

BE THE MVP OF YOUR MVS

MOVEMENT VITAL SIGNS WILL SAVE YOUR LIFE

Bo Babenko, DPT

MY STORY

It was a standard insurance form for freshman football camp. "Hey, Mom, what should I put for Dad?" In her thick Russian accent, I heard "diseased," which was odd despite my general knowledge, from the last time I saw him, that he was drinking a lot of alcohol and smoking a lot of cigarettes. "Wait, do you mean *deceased—like dead*?" "Yes." "Oh, when did that happen?"

To my shock, he had a heart attack seven years earlier, at age 41 and passed away; I thought they just separated, and he moved away.

Now, any distant hopes I'd harbored of seeing him again—of backyard catches or watching him cheering me on from the stands while I played quarterback—were gone for good.

Looking back, this was absolutely the catalyst for wanting to live my own healthy life and help other children not lose their parents from preventable diseases. I began to pursue career paths in working with the human body. After interning with chiropractors and orthopedic surgeons, and working as an emergency medical technician (EMT), athletic trainer, and personal trainer, I finally found my best fit in physical therapy. I felt I could make a huge difference in this field, which naturally blends the art of caring with the evidence-based science of healing. Unfortunately, as I became more and more exposed to the healthcare space, I became more and more skeptical and cynical of the systems in place to truly heal an individual.

I ended up naming my business FitCare Physiotherapy because I have found the concept of "FITness" to be the best way to avoid the healthCARE space. The current healthcare space is fantastic if you have a car accident and just want to survive, but not so good if you actually want to *thrive* in your physical body.

One of the most important things I see missing from the Physical Therapy profession is a push for an Annual Movement Screen. Just as dentists have pushed for twice-a-year checkups, we, as musculoskeletal experts, have discussed this concept for decades, but alas, there continues to be a lack of agreement about what this can look like.

We aren't being proactive. My favorite analogy with the current healthcare system is that we're relying on lifeguards when someone is in trouble in the water (getting sick and injured) when we would all be best served investing in a swimming instructor as early as possible to help us navigate the murky waters of life. Find that swimming instructor!

All that I find wrong with the medical system and fitness space is beyond this chapter. My frustration led me to create a podcast with a personal trainer buddy called "Demand Better," where we help people advocate for themselves to get more out of their care.

What we've noticed is the concept of *Movement* as one of the most essential ways that you can take control of your own health journey. What can you do today, once you put this book down, to demand better from your own body? I recommend focusing on your Movement Vital Signs.

Let's explore.

THE SKILL

UNDERSTANDING FUNCTIONAL MOVEMENTS AND MOVEMENT VITAL SIGNS

Functional movements are natural, everyday actions that use multiple joints and muscle groups working together. They include squatting (sitting and standing), hinging (bending at the hips), lunging (stepping forward or backward), pushing, pulling, carrying, and twisting. The stronger and more coordinated we are in controlling our bodies while we do them, the more efficiently and safely we can perform our daily activities.

Squat – Sitting down and standing up.

Hinge – Bending at the hips, like picking something off the floor.

Lunge – Stepping forward or backward, as in climbing stairs.

Push – Pressing something away, like opening a door.

Pull – Drawing something toward you, like pulling a rope.

Carry – Holding and moving objects, such as groceries or a suitcase.

Twist – Rotating the body, as in turning to grab something.

When you see your general doctor, they should be checking your blood pressure, cholesterol levels, and a number of other standard metrics that we can call "vital signs." We have these concepts for our cars, teeth, pets, mathematics (in school), and homes, but assessments are often missing with our movement. Movement vital signs assess how well your body performs functional movements. If you haven't heard "Movement is medicine," "Motion is lotion," and "Muscle is the organ of longevity," please allow me to introduce these concepts into your lexicon. These are the key principles to ensuring our bodies function optimally over a lifetime.

Whether you're an NFL player or an older adult trying to safely carry out daily activities, you'll be utilizing similar functional movements —but with different intensities and challenges. I'll focus on three essential goals for health and safety for anyone:

Controlling our body in space

Moving external loads

Pushing our lungs to work harder when we need

Achieving these goals requires us to focus on building strength, maintaining full joint motion, improving balance, and enhancing lung capacity.

Here's a bit of how I think about these and how they translate to **three key vital signs for longevity and health:**

1. Strength, especially grip strength and leg strength

2. Lung capacity/endurance

3. Flexibility/Full range of motion of our joints.

STRENGTH:

Strength is vital for maintaining functional independence, especially as we age. Grip and leg strength are particularly important because they can directly influence our ability to prevent falls—one of the most significant threats to health in older adults.

Functional strength should be thought of as our retirement fund for health. Most folks certainly begin to understand the power of compounding interest at some phase of their life (hopefully sooner than later, as investing $1000 at the age of 20 can turn into much more money than doing so at the age of 60). Muscle and strength work in a very similar way.

Keeping with the financial analogy, strength training is the closest thing we have to an eight percent yearly returning mutual fund or standard gold investment. All of the benefits of a stronger body would be exactly what you're looking for from a magic health pill—better resilience to any injury or accident, less likely to be sick, improved ability to go shopping or dance with your grandchild.

I've heard a litany of excuses over the years of why folks haven't included strength training in their exercise mix (don't want to look too bulky, not sure where to start, afraid of injury). These are all valid until you find a knowledgeable guide. No matter the rationale, I have to etch it in stone that avoiding strength training is like not putting any money into your retirement savings (no matter how old you are or when you plan to retire).

The cascade of benefits from having improved muscle mass are well documented including benefits to your hormones. As we age and begin dealing with issues like perimenopause (hormone loss), osteopenia (bone loss), or unwanted weight gain, your muscle mass could be the difference between many more vital years and needing assistance for basic activities like bathing and dressing oneself.

Here are some ways to assess strength: (please note that any pain with testing is a "red flag" and you should find a local health care provider who can properly assess what may be happening):

GRIP STRENGTH:

Dynamometer Test: A hand-held dynamometer is a device that shows how strong your grip is (costs about $25 on Amazon). You can easily assess your own baseline level and track it over time.

Hanging Test: The ability to hang from a bar tests endurance and grip stamina. How long can someone maintain their hold?

Suitcase Carry: This test bridges the gap between strength and function. Carrying heavy objects challenges both grip strength and overall body stability, offering a real-world application of grip with weight and need for balance.

LEG STRENGTH:

Single-Leg Stance: This assesses balance and stability, testing leg strength through the ability to hold a position on one leg. It reveals endurance and coordination in the lower body.

Leg Press: This is often done on gym machines. The leg press allows us to measure how much weight a person can push, reflecting strength through a full range of motion.

Squat with Weight: A squat is one of the most important functional movements. Whether simply getting up from a chair or for lifting heavy objects; it measures leg power and muscular endurance, coordination and balance, especially when performed with heavy weight.

LUNG CAPACITY/ENDURANCE- VO2 MAX

VO2 Max is a measure of how well we can bring oxygen into our bodies, and push carbon dioxide out. It reflects our cardiovascular fitness and aerobic endurance—essentially, how efficiently our heart, lungs, and muscles work together to deliver oxygen to our body during physical activity.

The ability to take in oxygen and expel carbon dioxide impacts everything from daily activities to athletic performance. The better your cardiovascular fitness, the easier it is to manage physical exertion, delay fatigue, and recover from strenuous activities.

Simple Endurance Test (Cooper Test):

The Cooper Test is a test to estimate VO2 max. The person runs as far as they can in 12 minutes on a flat, measured track. The total distance run is then used to estimate VO2 max based on a formula which we'll link to on our resource page.

The modified Cooper test is a variation and is adapted to allow walking or jogging instead of running, and the duration can be shortened to suit different fitness levels. The goal is to measure how far a person can move in the set time to estimate endurance and overall fitness.

Advanced Treadmill Test:

In a clinical or lab setting, VO2 max is often measured using a graded exercise test on a treadmill. The intensity increases gradually (by speed or incline) while oxygen consumption is monitored through a face mask or mouthpiece.

RANGE OF MOTION/JOINT FLEXIBILITY

As an orthopaedic and sports physiotherapist, one of the biggest takeaways I can share is to make sure we move our joints well and fully. This often gets glossed over. Arthritis, which is known as a "disease of modern living," we tend to think of as just from wear and tear. But it often comes from not moving fully, causing the joints to "rust up." Some of the most common surgeries in the US are knee and hip replacements. I believe (and it has been studied) that the more ability to move the hips and knees through their full range, the less chance of needing these surgeries.

In countries like China and India, achieving a deep squat is built into the culture for many activities for their entire lives, including eating, having a cup of coffee, and even using the toilet. These cultures tend to have almost no need for total knee or hip replacements, as has become a norm in the cultures where we're told to "not squat below 90 degrees." When I demonstrate the "ass to grass" squat, so many folks look at me like, "I could never do that," or "That hurts to even watch," which is one of the sadder aspects of my job on a daily basis. The phrase "ass to grass" refers to a technique in squatting where you lower your body so deeply that your hips come as close as possible to your heels, effectively bringing your "ass" close to the "grass." This is often known as a full range-of-motion (ROM) squat.

Hip and Knee: One great way to test your hip and knee range of motion, is with a squat. See how low you can go. On my chapter resource webpage there are links to work towards proper squat form.

Shoulder: One of the ways to test for shoulder range of motion is to see how far you can reach up behind your back. Can you touch your shoulder blades? Compare left to right. You can compare year to year.

The physical demands of an NFL player and your grandmother might seem worlds apart, but they actually follow the same principles—they just differ in scale. For a football player, powering through a 600-pound back squat tests strength and explosiveness. For your grandmother, rising from a chair might seem simple, but it's her version of a functional squat, requiring balance, coordination, and muscle strength.

Both tasks rely on the same muscles and movement patterns, emphasizing how foundational strength training and mobility exercises are for everyone, no matter their stage of life. The main difference is the intensity: NFL players train for peak performance, while your grandmother trains for daily life independence.

PRACTICAL EXERCISES FOR FUNCTIONAL STRENGTH

1. **Suitcase Carry: Strength and Stability** Imagine carrying a heavy bag through an airport—this movement assesses your grip strength, core stability, and overall body control.

   With one arm at a time, pick up a heavy object, like a dumbbell, kettlebell, or even a loaded bag, with one hand. Stand tall, keeping your shoulders level (don't lean toward the weight).

   Beginner: Use a lightweight and walk on flat ground.

   Intermediate: Increase the weight and distance or time

   Advanced: Try walking on uneven surfaces like grass or sand for an added challenge.

   A great number to aim for is to be able to carry half of your body weight with one hand for 90 seconds at a time—go as heavy as you can, rest 60 seconds between arms, and continue to work to get this stronger.

Make it a family ritual every Sunday morning, with everyone testing how much they can do. Perform this once a month if every week is not realistic.

2. **Single-Leg Stand: Balance and Stability** Test how long you can **stand on one leg.**

Beginner: Stand on one leg near a wall or chair for support. Can you hold for ten seconds?

Intermediate: Stand on one leg without support for 30 seconds.

Advanced: Stand on one leg, close your eyes, and hold. If you can get to 60 seconds on each leg, you probably do not need to do this test more than once a year. If you notice these numbers getting lower each year, it might be time to see a professional.

A lot of elderly folks have trouble getting to ten seconds, so the older we get the more important this vital sign becomes.

3. **Get up off the Ground.** How efficiently can you get up from the ground to a standing position from A to B? There is a strong correlation between this, fitness and survivability.

Yay, burpees! Some of you may know what a burpee exercise is. It's really an advanced way of getting up off the ground quickly, efficiently, and even protecting yourself from a fall. It's a great exercise. But essentially, your goal needs to be to get up any way you can.

How many times can you get up off the ground in over the course of two minutes? Eventually, as you practice, you'll find the most efficient way. You can also experiment with using one or even no arms.

Before you try any of these activities, you need to assess your ability to do so safely without risking injury. Back in the 90s, I recall this message during TV commercials when they promoted medications or some new weight loss regimen: "Check with your doctor before starting a new exercise program." I want to bring this concept back. So please check with your friendly neighborhood movement expert (best if they have some advanced degree like a DPT).

The list of possible ways to test your fitness can almost feel infinite, and these are just a few. But it seems the most important piece is finding something that makes sense to you and that you can stay consistent with. Creating accountability for yourself is *key*. This is a huge piece of personal training or group fitness classes for which you're more likely to show up and stay consistent. Find a challenge your whole family will take part in; perhaps you do this every Thanksgiving with your family, and the winner gets first dibs on the turkey or grandma's award-winning sweet potato casserole. Whatever your family fitness concept is, I encourage you to implement it as soon as you put this book down, and, personally, I would love to hear all about it. Shoot me an email here DrBo@fitcarephysio.com.

Here are some fun and bonding fitness habits that you can do with the kids in your life as a family or a class:

- Doing a family walk for ten minutes after every/most meal.
- Once a week garage gym sessions or a park "fitness" day where you can all play catch or do some form of movement.
- Hang test—who can hang the longest from a standard pull-up bar?
- Suitcase carry tests (one hand at a time)—who can carry the most weight as a percentage of their body weight? Ninety seconds is a nice way to test this per hand.
- Monthly grip strength challenge using a hand-held dynamometer

My son has only just turned two at the time of writing this, but I'm designing my workouts today and into the future to be able to play catch with him in the backyard the way I wish my father could've done with me. I also hope to instill in my son as he grows up, the concept of training hard and challenging himself in workouts so that when life gets hard physically and/or mentally—he will be more resilient. Who doesn't want to raise a mentally strong child? Find your *why* for training, and you'll be much more likely to stick with any game plan. It's up to you to figure out what program is sustainable for you and your family.

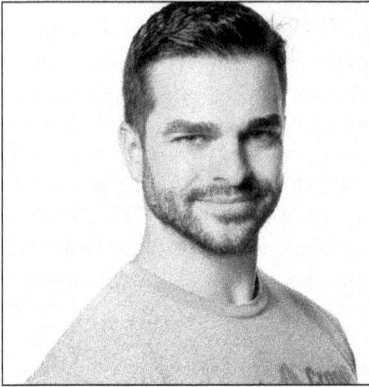

Dr. Bo Babenko, a passionate physical therapist, is dedicated to helping people maintain their physical abilities and avoid the injuries, surgeries, and medications that often sideline them unnecessarily. Inspired by the loss of his father to a heart attack at age 41, Bo has devoted his life to promoting choices that empower longevity and vitality.

Bo grew up in Brooklyn, New York, traveled the world as a private physiotherapist for a celebrity client, and ran a CrossFit gym in Dubai. He is now based in Erie, Colorado, with his dog Lexi, young son, and wonderful wife. Doctor Bo's mission is to keep people active and strong for life.

Bo runs FitCare Physiotherapy & Wellness, a practice built on the principle that fitness should be proactive, not reactive. Through in-person and online services, he helps clients relieve pain, build resilience, and feel stronger than ever. With 20 years of experience in strength and conditioning, Bo combines manual therapy, dry needling, breath work, and, most importantly, his clear and practical approach to navigating fitness and health. He's convinced the greatest tool he can provide is by clearing out all the medical and fitness system confusion his clients present with, to ultimately focus on a simple and sustainable way to get them 1% healthier every day.

Connect with Bo:

LinkedIn: https://www.linkedin.com/in/bobabenko

Instagram: @drbobabenko

Website: www.fitcarephysio.com

CHAPTER 23

NATURE MOVES

EXERCISE BEYOND CALORIES
AND HEART BEATS

Amanda A. Carpenter, DPT, CProT, CEAS

"What gets us into trouble is not what we don't know. It's what we know for sure that just ain't so."

~ Mark Twain

MY STORY

Exercising like crazy burned my energy but not my fat. I spent 20 years doing exercise all wrong, and as a professional, I didn't know any different.

"Make yourself comfortable. Put your sweatshirt back on, grab a bolster for under your legs." The instructor's voice grew louder as she approached me. "Do you want your feet covered up?" she asked, draping a blanket over them.

"Yes, please, I'd love that."

Thirty years ago, I would've never accepted such support. I believed I was strong enough to do everything myself, never asking for or accepting help.

Today, I'm different in many ways.

"Imagine walking through a meadow and coming upon a river. Bend down, touch the water, let it wash away what no longer serves you. Are you ready to let the river carry it downstream?" Her voice faded as I relaxed, drifting away from the room and the hardwood floor beneath me.

Gentle music played as the person next to me gathered their things. I decided to lay there in peace for a few more minutes—something I once wouldn't have allowed myself. Ah, it feels so good to just be. Nothing matters but this present moment.

I've come a long way from that awkward 13-year-old who believed she needed to be skinny to be likable, who believed she had to figure it all out on her own, who feared the spotlight and thought she had to be independent, never asking for help.

In this very building in 1991, I attended group aerobics. A repurposed textile factory on the Schroon River in Warrensburg, New York, built in the early 1800s. Three dollars for an hour of intense cardio. Some days, we used the Reebok step; other days we moved and grooved before lying on the floor for a glut and ab burn routine. My friend and I were the youngest in a class of about ten middle-aged women. Though not specified as women-only, there were no men.

I began intentional exercise in sixth grade; my intention was weight loss. Too young for organized sports, I found other ways to exercise. Despite being a poor swimmer, I attempted laps in my friend's pool. I never credited myself for the effort, rather criticizing my form and dismissing it as exercise because it wasn't sustained cardiovascular activity, which I was told was necessary for weight loss. Finding any way possible in the early 1990s to formally exercise without a gym was a challenge. I vaguely remember my muscle burn following a woman in a pink jumpsuit via a VHS calisthenics video in my living room. The light blue carpet scratching my skin.

My motivation stemmed from fear. Initially, I hated exercising but forced myself in an attempt to avoid being overweight like my older sister, who was teased. Additionally, my skinny friends received more attention from older boys. So many signs around me that indicated everything was better and easier for thinner girls.

That same 13-year-old also began dieting. After all, diet and exercise were the keys to a healthy weight. The early '90s trend was low-fat, allowing me to eat as much sugar as I wanted. All while exercising excessively just to maintain chubby. I guzzled fruit punch I made from a concentrate to fill my belly while avoiding butter, eggs, and most meats. As long as it was fat-free, I was fine, and calories in, less than calories out equals weight loss, right? Another misconception for another time.

I continued focusing on exercise and played organized sports in high school: volleyball, basketball, softball, and travel club volleyball. After practices or games, I walked my black lab, Odie, three miles. Despite sports, I woke early to work out on my stair stepper before school. Once I could drive, I awoke before sunrise, driving 30 minutes to the nearest Nautilus gym before school started at 8:02 a.m. This pattern continued into college, with at least one to two hours at the gym daily, and Billy Blanks Tae Bo® via VHS in the privacy of my dorm room. In grad school, I became a certified personal trainer, spending hours in the gym and exercising between clients. My drive was always the same: to lose or maintain my weight. The story I told myself was that exercise was good for me. I was healthy because of it, but the truth was I had a chronic, compulsive physiological need to exercise. Pushing myself to jog or walk five miles a day in addition to body weight-assisted exercises seven days a week, never allowing myself to rest unless something came up and I couldn't fit my workout in.

Exercise became an addiction fueled by the fear of weight gain. When I couldn't exercise, I was miserable. This misery stemmed from guilt and shame, not a lack of endorphins.

Now, I'm going to have to skip some meals. I'm never going to fit in the dress next week. No one will ever fall in love with me.

My passion for fitness led me to a career where I could incorporate it. I earned an undergraduate degree in health science and a master's in physical therapy, and became certified as a professional trainer (CProT), a personal trainer with a medical license. As an overachiever, I eventually went on to pursue a Doctorate in Physical Therapy and moved back to upstate New York to open Carpenter Physical Therapy, an outpatient orthopedic practice closely tied to athletics and fitness. This passion project had me working 60-70 hours per week, encroaching on my exercise time.

Two years without serious exercise left me exhausted, overweight, with aching joints and a pounding headache. I believed returning to regular exercise was the solution. Exhausted, tired, and wired, I wished for more hours in the day, yet I awoke at 5:00 a.m. to work out before my ten-hour workday.

My body longed for rest and ached after simply walking the dog.

You're exhausted because you've put on some extra weight; come on, step it up. More weight gain will cause you to have less energy. It's just a little muscle soreness because you haven't worked out in so long.

Fear drove me to push myself even harder despite feeling terrible. Fueled by adrenaline, caffeine, and the pressure to cure myself with exercise, I believed all I needed was to get through the delayed onset muscle soreness stage, and everything would be okay. Until one day, walking the dog became too painful and exhausting. My body ached from a simple two-and-a-half-mile walk. I recall coming home, lying on the floor, unable to take another step.

What is happening? I've always exercised my way back to feeling good. Something is different; something is wrong. I can't do this anymore.

Eventually, I was diagnosed with an acute tick-borne illness. (Read my story in *Holistic Mental Health: Calm, Clear, and In Control for the Rest of Your Life, Volume 2* by Laura Mazzotta)

My body was massively inflamed. Not only did I lack the energy to exercise, but when I tried, my body couldn't recover. I harmed myself by breaking down my body when it lacked the resources to recover. Strenuous exercise is contraindicated with acute infections.

It took three years to regain my health. My self-care practices, including exercise, look very different today. I haven't worked out in a formal gym since 2008. My physical activity is different than it was 25-30 years ago, not because I'm older, but because I now know better. Instead of heavy cardiovascular or strength training, I walk my dogs three to five miles daily and attend restorative yoga classes. Living in the Southern Adirondack Mountains, I get outside daily, a key to mitochondrial health. My activities consist of walking, hiking, swimming, kayaking, and snowshoeing with my husband, friends, and dogs. We get plenty of daily outdoor physical activity with sunshine and cold exposure.

Now, lying on this same hardwood floor of the old textile factory over 30 years later, awakening from Savasana at the end of my 90-minute restorative yoga class, I send love and compassion to that awkward 13-year-old who believed she needed to be anything other than her authentic self, who thought she needed to spend time indoors suffering and sweating, and who followed mainstream exercise and diet trends. I have so much gratitude for the drive and determination of that 18 y/o who followed her obsession with exercise and made it into a career.

Having spent 25 years in healthcare as a physical therapist, 15 of those focused on holistic and foundational health, I've discovered two very important keys to health and vitality:

1. Limiting beliefs drive the habits that lead to health decline.

2. Often the mind obstructs the body's ancient wisdom.

We don't need more exercise, working out alone under artificial lights while breathing recycled air. Our bodies are actually craving outdoor physical activity in a state of joy while connecting with others.

Have you been trying to exercise, but it's not quite working for you? I've got some things for you to consider in the section below.

Do the best you can until you know better. Then, when you know better, you do better.

~ Maya Angelou

THE SKILL

The human body needs physical activity, not always exercise. It has been said that sitting is the new smoking, and inefficient physical activity can negatively impact health. The human body thrives on physical activity, not just exercise. While many use these terms interchangeably, they differ significantly in how they affect our physiology. Let's clarify this distinction.

Exercise involves repeated movements aimed at improving strength or endurance, pushing the body to a point of breakdown. This stress triggers inflammation, prompting a healing response that strengthens muscles. For instance, doing squats to muscle fatigue signals stress, leading to muscle repair and growth, provided the body has a healthy inflammatory response.

For effective healing, certain conditions are essential:

1. Adequate deep sleep for this tissue repair. https://leadingwithvitality.com/sleephabitsplaybook

2. A proper and adequate inflammatory response.

3. Sufficient nutrients from whole foods for tissue repair. This requires healthy digestion.

Each of these conditions hinges on a regulated nervous system, crucial for overall health. Heart-focused breathing, a technique brought to us and researched by the HeartMath™ Institute, is a foundational and simple way to begin to support nervous system regulation.

Check out this video on heart-focused breathing:
https://tinyurl.com/mv6ra5ke

For additional self-regulation techniques:
https://leadingwithvitality.com/optin1659368887765

Previously, cardiovascular exercise was thought to improve heart efficiency through repetitive stress. However, the HeartMath™ Institute's research highlights the heart's recovery quality after stress, like exercise or emotional events, as a key to health. Emotional regulation is a greater contributing factor to cardiovascular health than repetitive cardiovascular exercise for the sake of keeping the heart rate elevated for prolonged periods.

According to Merriam-Webster, exercise involves the regular or repeated use of a body part or exertion to develop and maintain physical fitness. The key difference between exercise and physical activity lies in the intensity and focus of stress on the body.

Physical activity refers to any movement of the body that requires energy expenditure. It includes a wide range of activities, from everyday tasks like walking, gardening, and cleaning to more structured forms like playing sports or dancing. Unlike exercise, which is often planned and repetitive with the goal of improving fitness, physical activity encompasses all movement that contributes to energy expenditure and overall health.

Physical activity is essential for health and vitality, primarily because it aids in lymphatic drainage. The lymphatic system, which removes waste from the body, lacks a direct mechanical pump. Instead, it relies on proper diaphragm movement during breathing and the body's physical movement to function effectively. Physical activity is also a way to move and nourish the joints, improve and enhance blood flow, and discharge excess energy from the nervous system.

The human body is designed to move in dynamic ways, such as crawling, climbing, scrambling, hiking, reaching, pushing, pulling, and lifting. These movements can be referred to as primal movements involved in physical activity. Turning these movements into activities might improve fitness more effectively than modern exercises that repeatedly stresses joints. Can you recall the challenge of the crab walk or bear crawl in elementary school?

Physical activity provides the primary benefits that the body needs for health and vitality. Many physical activities occur outdoors, carrying additional benefits related to natural light exposure, grounding, and the impact of the colors of nature on the body's chemistry.

Here are some examples of physical activity:

- Dancing (my favorite)
- Jumping on a trampoline (another personal favorite; yup, I have one in my yard)
- Playing tag
- Hiking
- Bear crawling and crab walking
- Swimming/playing in the water
- Any type of sport

YOUR THOUGHTS IMPACT WHAT HAPPENS INSIDE THE BODY DURING EXERCISE AND ACTIVITY.

The human body was designed to run as an escape from predators. Therefore, at its root, it doesn't understand the difference between exercising on a treadmill and running from a bear. The intention behind why you are moving your body sets the foundation for what will happen to the biochemistry. Fear isn't a healthy motivator. Are you dreading the gym but telling yourself that the exercise is necessary for good health? Is there a discipline in getting yourself to exercise or move your body? What are your thoughts while you are exercising? Again, fear shifts the chemistry away from vitality. Is your mind in the future? Are you worried about getting everything done and reviewing your to-do list? If your mind is in a place of fear, either rehashing the past or dreading the future, your body doesn't really know the difference between exercise for fitness and the primal state of fear and the need to escape.

The greatest benefit comes when we exercise with a healthy mindset. Setting an intention to move the body in a healthy, self-nourishing way sets the stage for a beneficial shift in chemistry. Staying present in the moment while feeling a renewing emotion is a great focus. Presence appears to be more fundamental to physical activity than exercise, perhaps due to the repetitive, trance-like nature of exercise.

EXERCISING FOR THE WRONG REASONS WON'T GIVE YOU THE GREATEST BENEFIT.

As I previously mentioned, fear is not a healthy motivator and will hijack the benefits of your exercise routine. The motivation behind your movement is extremely important. Forcing yourself to go to the gym in the name of prevention will not give you the benefits that physical activity has to offer. Consider prioritizing physical activity time with your friends (even the furies) and your family. Joy greatly benefits the human body in numerous ways and is the natural state for both children and dogs.

SOMETIMES WHAT THE BODY NEEDS IS TO SLOW DOWN WHILE MOVING.

The autonomic nervous system has two sides: the parasympathetic and the sympathetic. The sympathetic nervous system often gets a bad reputation as the fight or flight response; however, this is not entirely true. The sympathetic nervous system is our body's gas pedal, the energy consumption state; it occurs when the body is in the state of doing. Doing can be in the form of thinking or physical movement. The parasympathetic nervous system, otherwise known as the rest and digest system, is our body's brake. Heart rate determines the difference between the sympathetic and parasympathetic nervous system. Exercise and activity that elevates the heart rate use energy, while gentle activity that lowers the heart rate recharges the body. This is exactly why restorative yoga is now part of my routine. Restorative yoga practices, as well as tai chi, are gentle forms of physical activity in a low heart rate state that can be incredibly recharging. Be aware of whether your routine depletes you or renews you and exactly what your body needs

THE SOUND AROUND YOU AND THE MUSIC YOU LISTEN TO CAN ALSO HAVE AN IMPACT ON YOUR BODY'S NERVOUS SYSTEM AND RESPONSE TO ACTIVITY.

Listening to stimulating music can elevate your heart rate while listening to gentle, relaxing music can aid your body in shifting toward a recharging state. Check out this intentional music to relax and recharge: https://signup.iah.fit/crystal-serenity

Physical activity in the form of dynamic movement is a necessary foundation of health. Exercise does count as activity, but as we discussed several factors need to be considered for the greatest benefit. True health and vitality come not from disciplined, isolated exercise routines under artificial conditions but from joyful, spontaneous physical activity that connects us with others and the natural world. Remember, the body needs recharging to benefit from exercise, so prioritize how you spend your activity time. When it comes to caring for your body, don't let the outside world drown out your inner wisdom.

Much Love,

Amanda

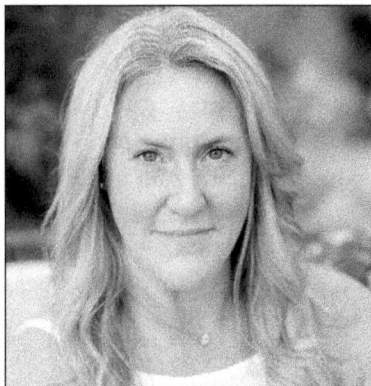

Dr. Amanda A. Carpenter, PT, CProT, CEAS, is the visionary CEO of iah.fit, a groundbreaking wellness platform that seamlessly integrates sacred wisdom with modern technology and science. Through transformative music, Heart-Centered AI™ guidance, and powerful visual art, iah.fit promotes holistic well-being and elevates human performance and vitality.

With a Doctorate in Physical Therapy and over two decades of expertise in human performance, Amanda has been a pioneer in integrating mind-body practices, heart coherence, and biofield enhancement into personalized wellness solutions. Her career is dedicated to empowering individuals to achieve optimal health and vitality.

Amanda's mission is to guide people back to their true selves, fostering trust in their bodies, cultivating deep human connections, and empowering individuals to unlock their superpowers. She understands the importance of daily foundational routines that blend nature and technology to create a life beyond one's wildest dreams.

Residing in a forest community in the Adirondack Mountains with her husband and two yellow labs, Amanda maintains her health with daily outdoor walks and regular sunlight and cold exposure. She also enjoys rejuvenating on the beaches of Aruba, embracing the lifestyle she inspires her clients to build.

Connect with Amanda:

Join my private community:
https://amandaacarpenter.mn.co/users/onboarding/plans

Facebook: https://www.facebook.com/amandaacarpenter

LinkedIn: https://www.linkedin.com/in/amanda-a-carpenter/

SLEEP, REPAIR, AND RECHARGE

"People say, 'I'm going to sleep now,' as if it were nothing. But it's really a bizarre activity. 'For the next several hours, while the sun is gone, I'm going to become unconscious, temporarily losing command over everything I know and understand. When the sun returns, I will resume my life."

~ George Carlin

SLEEP, REPAIR, AND RECHARGE:

AN OVERVIEW

The quote on the previous page, by comedian George Carlin captures the oddness—and the profundity—of sleep. Sleep may seem like "switching off" for the night, but it's a vital process that restores and powers our entire body. It's an unseen process, yet critical to everything we do.

We hear a lot about quantity of sleep—how many hours we should be getting... but not enough about quality—how well we sleep during those hours.

The sleep pillar chapters will delve into this more:

One chapter provides an overview of quality sleep fundamentals and what it truly means to embrace restorative rest.

The other highlights the vital role of nasal breathing, explaining how it helps ensure steady oxygen flow, balances the nervous system, and prevents disruptions common with sleep-disordered breathing. It's one of the most effective practices to enhance your sleep quality—and, ultimately, your life quality.

SLEEP GOALS

- **Duration:** Seven to nine hours (of actual sleep- not time awake in bed). Find your sweet spot of how long works best for you.
- **Quality:** Cycling through deep sleep, rem sleep, few awakenings, steady oxygen, and lowered heart rate help you wake feeling rested.
- **Consistency:** Bedtime/wake time helps to set the day's rhythm and improves sleep efficiency.

SLEEP REGULATING PROCESSES

Process S—Sleep/Wake Homeostasis:

The longer you stay awake, the more likely you'll feel sleepy (sleep pressure).

Process C— Circadian Clock:

Our internal clock is synchronized with Earth's 24-hour rotation cycle.

The timing of our internal circadian clock is influenced by external cues:

- Light
- Temperature
- Noise
- Eating/drinking patterns
- Surrounding environment quality
- Exercise
- Social interaction schedule
- Mental health/mindset
- Mental stimulation
- Nutrients
- Medications

Intentionally designing our day and environment to enhance their influence on our sleep is incredibly impactful. Many are in our control, allowing us the opportunity to proactively and quickly start building lasting power habits.

SHIFTWORK AND TACTICAL HOURS

Sometimes, due to essential responsibilities, you can't sleep the recommended hours and in the most supportive environment for your needs. But do the best you can—use your fresh understanding of sleep science to build on your existing skills, and continue to learn how to make it work best for you.

Focus on creating a consistent routine, reducing disruptions, and prioritizing quality over quantity. Experiment with strategies like *strategic napping* (used by the military), managing light exposure, and using relaxation techniques. These small adjustments can help you maximize your sleep and deep rest opportunities, and support your overall health and performance.

WHEN SLEEP ISN'T POSSIBLE

There are times when, no matter how hard we try, sleep just won't come. The recently coined term *Non Sleep Deep Rest* (NSDR) involves techniques that help you get close to being in a deep sleep physiological state, without actually sleeping. While not a substitute for sleep, they can be a powerful ally to help you attain a restorative state.

The best strategy we know of today is *Yoga Nidra* also known as "yogic sleep". It's an ancient guided meditation practice with the goal of reaching a deep state of relaxation while remaining conscious and aware.

Our ultimate goal is to give our bodies the time, space and resources to reach a restorative state during which we can recharge and repair. Sleep is the key and ultimate strategy to achieve this. Engaging in NSDR techniques can complement this process, helping to foster relaxation and restoration when enough or quality sleep is disrupted.

CHAPTER 24

SLEEP: OUR NIGHT SHIFT

RECHARGING, REPAIRING, AND BUILDING RESILIENCE WHILE WE REST

Ilana Zablozki-Amir MD, dipABMPR, IFMCP
with Patrick Nardulli, USN (Ret)

"Sleep is not an option; it is a necessity. We are in a sleep crisis in America, and it is time to take sleep seriously."

~ William Dement, Sleep Researcher

MY STORY

I never thought much about sleep. In college and medical school, I was the master of all-nighters before tests and project deadlines. I worked best under pressure. I did well and really don't remember "crashing" the following day.

Then came my medical residency—definitely not sleep-friendly. There were 24-hour shifts that turned into almost 36 hours of being awake to catch up on notes and meetings, and this happened multiple days per week.

I also loved to socialize and was often in FOMO (fear of missing out) mode. One of my anthems was Jon Bon Jovi's *I'll Sleep When I'm Dead*.

My ability to function well on short bursts of sleep served me very well in the most blessed years when I got to cuddle with my kids at night and readily be there for them when they needed — to change the sheets when they accidentally wet the bed, to tell them stories to help them fall back asleep after a nightmare or to welcome them as they came to join my husband and me in our bed. I loved every second!

It really wasn't until I started delving into understanding the foundational principles of health that I began to grasp the profound importance of sleep. We're designed with an inherent blueprint for renewal, and sleep is the key to unlocking it.

Sleep is the irreplaceable time to reboot, recharge, repair—and even clean. While we sleep, our bodies initiate these essential mechanisms: hormones recalibrate, tissues regenerate, memories solidify, and immune defenses strengthen. During deep sleep is the only time the brain gets to clear out toxins and waste that accumulate throughout the day. Sleep is far from a passive state; it's a powerful, active process that upholds every aspect of our health. Recognizing its role shifts sleep from a nice-to-have to an absolute necessity—one that directly determines our resilience and vitality.

Inherently we're made to sleep. Our lives depend on it. So why is it difficult for so many? Some kind of difficulty sleeping is one of the most common concerns I hear from patients, acquaintances, friends, and family. As a physician, it's not always easy to solve

I, too, have my own difficulties sleeping. Since becoming a mother (and even before, from being the doctor on call) I tend to sleep in a vigilant state— subconsciously on alert for any potential needs or threats around me. That's my speed bump to sleep. Some nights, I get great quality sleep, and others, my on-guard brain wakes me way too early, well before the birds start chirping.

But what I've come to understand is that despite this, the quality of my sleep—and of everyone's—ultimately rests on the choices we make throughout the day and the environment we create for ourselves at night. As I'm mindful of this, I can subjectively and objectively (via my health metric tracking ring) see the impact.

Knowing what I know now, I still wouldn't have given up those "mommy moments," but I certainly would've prioritized family sleep habits, focusing on quality as much as quantity—habits my boys could rely on through the demands of college, long workdays, and all stages of life, especially when sleep is so readily sacrificed and easily interrupted.

One of our *Healthy for Life* authors, Patrick Nardulli, USN (Ret.), who provided us with invaluable wisdom about our nervous system in chapter 17, is also a highly experienced sleep educator and coach. He works in close collaboration with leading sleep scientists, contributing to sleep research for the US military, and is the lead author of sleep curricula currently used in training operational forces in the US Navy. He has helped me formulate the essential messages of this chapter.

THE SKILL

EMBRACING SLEEP

If you think about it, sleep isn't just downtime. We don't just close after hours like a small shop. We're a complex operational system, like a massive supermarket, essential factory, and national security department all in one. Each has its own "night shift," and we have ours, which is very active while we're sleeping.

Our "sleep-shift" team has limited hours to optimize operations and needs ideal conditions to be efficient; without enough time or resources, essential work is missed, which then impacts the rhythm of the next day. For us, this means creating an environment and routine that allows sleep to work at its best.

Did You Know? According to the Centers for Disease Control, one in three adults doesn't get enough sleep regularly. But what does "enough sleep" actually mean, and why is it so elusive? And what are the repercussions? The answers, surprisingly, go well beyond what you may expect

WHAT DOES ENOUGH SLEEP MEAN?

It means enough sleep to do what our night shift, the "sleep-shift" needs to do.

During sleep, our body and brain cycle through different stages, each with their own responsibilities. The stages that nature designed for us are called our *Sleep Architecture*.

NREM sleep (Non-REM): It has three stages: light, deeper, and deep. Deep sleep is where the heavy lifting of restoration occurs. During this phase, human growth hormone is released, tissue is repaired, muscle is built, and our immune system is strengthened. The brain uses this time to clean house, clearing out metabolic waste and setting us up for greater mental clarity.

REM (Rapid Eye Movement) sleep: The stage during which we dream, process and organize what we've learned and experienced earlier in the day, secure memories, and process emotions.

We naturally cycle through these stages 4-5 times per night (each cycle takes approximately 90 minutes). We need to allot enough time to allow ourselves go through each cycle enough times, so we don't shortchange the processes that are indispensable for physical recovery, resilience, mental well-being, and our peak productivity the next day.

Research has found that it takes about 7-9 hours to effectively cycle through. Each person tends to have a sweet spot within this range after which they feel and function at their best. Children and teens actually need more, depending on the stage of growth and development they are in.

What are the repercussions of not getting proper quality sleep?

Think of sleep like a bank account. Every time you miss out on sleep, you "borrow" rest from your body, creating what scientist's call sleep debt. The more you miss, the more you owe. Unlike regular debt, you can't pay it all back in one go, like sleeping in on the weekend. Instead, your body needs steady, quality sleep over time to catch up.

If you regularly miss out on sleep, your body builds up this debt, which can lead to fatigue, poor focus, mood issues, struggling memory, daytime drowsiness, slower reaction time, and host of longer-term health concerns including harder to control blood sugar and blood pressure, inflammation and lowered immunity. It then becomes a vicious cycle, as many of these same factors influence the quality of our sleep.

There is also an additional danger—as people become more sleep-deprived, they become less aware that they're impaired.

Notable fact: one of the ways to know if you are in sleep debt is if you fall asleep within fewer than five minutes of your head hitting the pillow.

WHY DOES A GOOD THOROUGH SLEEP SEEM SO ELUSIVE?

A good, thorough sleep seems elusive for many reasons, most of which have deep roots in our culture and daily habits. Society often doesn't prioritize sleep as a fundamental aspect of health and productivity. Instead, we're conditioned to believe that maximizing time awake and staying busy defines success.

When we constantly occupy our minds, we're directly impacting our sleep physiology, making it harder for the brain and body to enter the deep, restorative phases of sleep. This pressure affects everyone, from kids to adults, where performance becomes a priority over rest.

And the societal undervaluing of sleep sends a powerful, often subtle message: rest isn't as essential as productivity. Yet, the truth is, sleep is as vital as any other health habit—perhaps even more so—because it recharges us in ways that impact everything else we do.

EACH OF US HAS OUR OWN UNIQUE SET OF REASONS THAT MAY IMPACT THE QUALITY OF OUR SLEEP.

Prioritizing Sleep

For some people, **lack of awareness about sleep's true importance,** leading them to neglect it entirely.

For others, the **demands of work, home, and family can stretch late into the night**—whether intentionally or not—causing them to stay up long past the point when their bodies are practically begging for rest. And the pressure can weigh on our minds long after we've closed our eyes.

Philosophically, sleep reveals our vulnerability; while awake, we maintain a sense of control, but surrendering that control during sleep can be uncomfortable. This dynamic may reflect **a subconscious fear of**

embracing sleep, and a cause for some to procrastinate going to bed, even when they have the opportunity to.

"Revenge bedtime procrastination" refers to the behavior of **delaying sleep in order to reclaim personal time that feels lost during the day** due to work or other responsibilities. People may stay up late, engaging in activities like scrolling through social media, watching TV, or pursuing hobbies, all in an attempt to enjoy some "me time" after a busy day. This phenomenon highlights the struggle between the desire for rest and the need for personal fulfillment, often leading to a cycle of sleep deprivation and fatigue.

Staying Asleep

If you ask ten people about their sleep challenges, you might hear eleven different answers. Snoring partners, chronic pain, frequent bathroom trips, racing thoughts, hot flashes, monthly hormone fluctuations, waking up for no reason, digestive discomfort, nightmares—these are all common struggles. Some may be from health imbalances and diagnosed conditions, and some could also be from side effects of medications. Sometimes addressing these are simple, and sometimes they require more nuanced solutions.

Sleep Saboteurs That Are More Readily In Our Control

Environment: Elements such as types and times of light exposure, including blue light from digital screens, temperature, noise, and the comfort of our sleeping arrangements, can significantly affect our ability to fall asleep and stay asleep.

Food and Drink: What we eat and drink (including high sugar foods, excessive caffeine, and alcohol) and when we consume it have a very strong influence. For example, consuming sugary foods, especially close to bedtime, can lead to a quick spike in blood sugar followed by a rapid drop, or "crash." The body interprets this sudden drop as a potential threat, prompting a stress response to stabilize energy levels. The body essentially shifts into a "survival mode," which disrupts the natural sleep cycle and makes it harder to fall back into a deep, restful sleep.

Stress: Few realize that not balancing our stress during the day and surrounding ourselves with stressful news and social situations in the evening, when its time time to wind down before sleep, are very real and strong sleep saboteurs.

When we're in a stressful situation, our key stress hormone—cortisol—rises.

But the effects of cortisol aren't limited to the moment of stress. Excess amounts linger in the blood until the body is ready and able to clear it. It can take hours. The more intense the stress, the longer it takes. Your body can't rest well when cortisol is high. It has a natural tendency to inhibit melatonin, our sleep hormone. Have you ever wondered why so many people use melatonin supplements to sleep? Intentionally using calming practices throughout the day (in our Nervous System Regulation Pillar, you'll find some key skills) helps keep cortisol in check, making it easier to relax at night.

Something to consider: The stressors of social media, such as social comparisons, the need for validation, and the overwhelming flow of information, also lead to an increase in the level of cortisol in our blood. If you're on social media close to bed, especially if you're a "doom-scroller" (continuously scrolling through distressing content) you're at inherent risk for doomed quality sleep.

HOW CAN WE USE THIS INFORMATION FOR OUR BENEFIT?

First, don't stress about it. Most people miss out on a good night's sleep here and there. If that happens to you, periodically, its fine. Sometimes it's not in our control, no sense worrying. But when one day starts turning into two or three days in a row, or multiple times a week, then it's time to take action.

In chapter one, I discussed the importance of Proactive Prevention, emphasizing the need to focus on what we can control rather than placing blame or surrendering to circumstances.

If quality sleep is your goal (hopefully by reading up to this point, it is):

Step 1: Identify which of these factors make sleep elusive for you. Likely a few.

Step 2: Reflect on which are in your immediate control and which may take a while to be able to address if at all.

Step 3: Once you understand what is relevant to you, and in which areas you can readily make a difference, you can take meaningful action with a *Proactive Sleep Action Plan.*

IMPLEMENTING A PROACTIVE SLEEP ACTION PLAN—A BRIEF OVERVIEW

A. Prioritize the Pillars:

Proactively and consistently implement strategies within all five *Healthy for Life* Pillars. Nutrition, hydration, nature, environmental quality, stress regulation, fitness and energy flow, and sleep prioritization all impact sleep. In other words, when you prioritize your daily actions, improved sleep will ultimately follow.

B. Recognize Your Risks:

Understand your risk factors and red flags for poor-quality sleep and sleep debt. Here are some key questions to ask yourself (and your children).

Sleep Self-Assessment:

- Are you consistently getting seven to nine hours of sleep (more for kids and teens)?
- Do you wake up feeling rested and alert, or are you often tired and sluggish unless you sleep more?
- Do you experience daytime sleepiness or rely on caffeine or naps to stay awake?
- Can you fall asleep easily, or do you struggle to wind down?
- How quickly do you "pass out" when your head hits the pillow?
- Do you snore or have you been told you gasp or stop breathing in your sleep?
- Do you use medications or supplements to help you sleep?
- Do you support your circadian rhythm with morning sunlight and limit blue light at night?
- Is your sleep environment dark, cool, and quiet?
- Are you often exposed to screens or blue light before bed?

C. Understand Your Terrain:

Assess objectively what's happening inside you.

What you can do for yourself:

Sleep Trackers: Use a credible sleep tracker (ring, watch, or strap) to gain insights into your sleep architecture, duration, stress levels, and body temperature changes. This objective information could be invaluable for understanding your sleep quality, as just relying on feeling rested alone, may not reflect the full picture.

What you can discuss with your practitioner:

Sleep Studies: Obtain a sleep study from your doctor, either in a lab or at home, to diagnose disorders like sleep apnea or narcolepsy. Keep in mind that these studies usually capture just one night of data.

What else could be contributing:

Lab testing can help you see what role your overall health and nutrition may be playing in affecting your sleep. For example:

Hormone levels: Imbalances in hormones such as cortisol (the stress hormone), melatonin (the sleep hormone), testosterone, progesterone, estrogen, and thyroid.

Nutrient levels: Vitamin D, B vitamins, iron, magnesium, protein/ amino acids, and essential fats, among others.

Metabolic Markers: Inflammation, blood sugar control, kidney or liver issues, blood cell count.

Food sensitivities: Can interfere with sleep quality, triggering symptoms that make it difficult for the body to relax and maintain restful sleep.

Gut Microbiome: Can provide insights into how the gut-brain connection may influence sleep, as gut bacteria play a role in making neurotransmitters (the brain's chemical messengers).

D. Build Your Toolbox and Team:

One of the most important tools, or skills, for sleep is to understand how to create a **Sleep Supportive Day**:

1. Reframe: It starts with framing/reframing our perspective on sleep. Sleep isn't a sign of weakness; it's an essential human need. Ditch fears around "losing time" to sleep. Think of it as your personal recharge to allow for a more resilient, productive, smarter, and healthier day to come.

2. Book End: Next is prioritizing time. Plan your day so you can spend seven to nine hours in bed, not just falling asleep but staying asleep. Count back from when you need to wake up—if you're up at 6 a.m., aim to be asleep by 11 p.m. Creating a wind-down routine of 30-60 minutes can help signal to your body that it's time for rest.

Interesting Fact: Sleep experts have found that consistent wake and sleep times train your body and brain to be efficient between those hours. Even though some people love spontaneity and to play things by ear, our bodies naturally gravitate towards routines and structure. The more you give it familiarity, the less guesswork it has to do.

"Book-ending" the day with specific actions tied to these times—your personalized wind-down routine at night and a wake-up routine in the morning help these become ingrained habits.

3. Cue the Clock: Your body has an internal clock, known as the Circadian Clock, which keeps your sleep-wake cycle in sync with the natural 24-hour day. This is a circadian rhythm. A small part of your brain, the suprachiasmatic nucleus (SCN), serves as the control center for this cycle, helping your body respond to natural light and dark. Light in the morning signals your brain to wake up and prepare for activity, while evening darkness helps it wind down and prepare for sleep.

Interesting Fact: Nearly every cell in your body has its own "clock," controlled by this central master clock in the brain! These cellular clocks regulate essential functions like hormone release, body temperature, and digestion. Together, they create a coordinated rhythm that affects everything from alertness to appetite.

External cues, called "zeitgebers" (meaning "time-givers" in German), help regulate this internal circadian clock. Light is the most important one. In addition to light, temperature, noise, eating/drinking timing, surrounding environment quality, exercise timing, social interaction schedule, and mental stimulation are some of the most impactful and most in our control.

Remember that a good night's sleep starts in the morning.

Intentionally creating a "circadian-supportive environment" day and night can be the most powerful step you can take to set yourself up for quality sleep. On our resource link, we have a step-by-step guide to help you do this. And here's the first step to get you started: Follow Nature's Light Rhythms: **Follow Nature's Light Rhythms**

"Light is the most powerful cue for our circadian clock. It sets the timing for our sleep, metabolism, and overall health"

~ Satchin Panda, Circadian Scientist

- **Bright Days:** Start your day with natural light—open your blinds or step outside within an hour of waking to set your internal clock. Afternoon tip: If you work inside, take a daylight break.
- **Dim Evenings:** Think sunset! Go out and enjoy it. Use warmer, dimmer lights and avoid harsh overhead lighting. Blue light-blocking glasses can help reduce any screen light exposure.
- **Dark Nights:** Consider using blackout curtains and cover any small lights from appliances and gadgets.

Add a cooler bedroom temperature, quiet and comfort and you've begun to set yourself up for quality restorative sleep.

Building/Recruiting your Team:

As you learn lots more about how to take the actions we've outlined here and others, learning how to practically, implement them is the key to making the changes that will support your goal of good sleep with minimal to no debt. Engage the trusted people that can help support your goals: family, friends, physical, psychological and complementary therapists, sleep coaches, etc. They can be invaluable for your progress. And ultimately in how you guide the kids under your care.

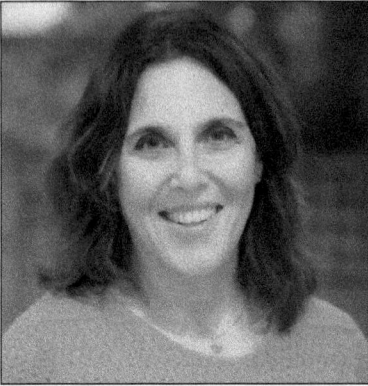

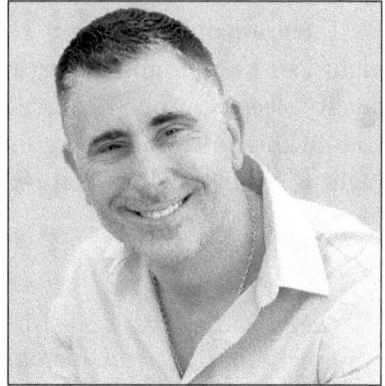

For full author bios for **Dr. Ilana Zablozki-Amir** and **Patrick Nardulli**, please see chapters 1 and 17

CHAPTER 25

BREATHLESS

THE LOST ART OF NASAL BREATHING

Najwa Jaber, DDS

"By the laws of average, you will take 670 million breaths in your lifetime. Maybe you'd like to take a few million more?"

~James Nestor

MY STORY

When your breath owns your smile...

...little did I know, it did.

In October 1974, my brother was a second-year medical student in Toulouse, France. He called home and pressed my parents to send me to his professor for an evaluation of my unsightly underbite—his main concern.

I was eight years old and had just started ballet classes, which my doctor suggested to stabilize my gait because I was known to be clumsy. My dance teacher, a stern Russian-French woman, would send unfriendly letters to my parents about their lack of attention to my health (untrue) because of ongoing upper respiratory infections.

Severe bad breath landed me at several ear, nose, and throat doctors (ENTs) and gastroenterologists without much improvement. Everyone seemed to doubt my abilities and my future success.

My parents put me on a flight from Dakar, Senegal, my first time on an airplane, to Toulouse, France, via Paris. I remember sobbing as I boarded that plane. Two days later, I was evaluated by a craniofacial surgeon, my brother's professor, who quickly determined my issue was my underdeveloped jaws and that I didn't need surgical intervention. Less than a week later, I was on my way back to Africa with upper and lower retainer-like appliances to be worn 24/7 which had to be activated once a week for the next three years of my life.

One day, in midsummer of 1977, at the age of 11, I returned home from my last dentist appointment and announced to my parents and the twenty-member family I lived with: " I no longer had to wear my retainers anymore!". Oh yes! I forgot to mention that I used to walk down to my dentist alone every Wednesday at 1 p.m. for a retainer activation and check-up. We were living in different times then.

I no longer had an underbite, my lips were better supported and sealed, my jawline was more pleasing, my sleep was no longer restless, and most of all, I had stopped bedwetting—and not because I was getting older!

Fast forward 46 years—It's the Covid era in the US—a ten-week lockdown! What better time to dive into the unknown and explore a new field of debate: the breath! Who would've imagined something so primitive and primal to life, essential to any living creature of the animal kingdom, was becoming a hot topic? *And it's related to our jaws?*

I received a random email one day from a large dental supply company venturing into education. They were offering a free introductory class about dentistry and obstructive sleep apnea. I quickly welcomed that opportunity to feel active and productive during a quarantine. I signed up for the class remotely, and for the next eight hours, I was glued to my desktop, getting educated on the subject that most of us don't ever think twice about—breathing!

As a dentist with 20 years of experience, I was now inspired to become a true stomatologist, a physician of the mouth (also known as the oral cavity) and the structure of the skull. What an opportunity for learning, growth, and healing it was! And it continues to be.

DENTISTRY TODAY IS BREATHTAKING

During our virtual session, hundreds of dentists from around the world received an incredible amount of researched-backed information. We explored topics like evolution, physiology, medical history, and cultural behaviors, which opened up a whole new way of thinking beyond traditional dentistry. It felt like I stepped through a massive gateway into a new world where healthcare providers are responsible not just for treatments but for staying informed, sharing, and applying new knowledge to help their patients.

Learning to identify signs of breathing issues just by looking at facial features in children and adults, and their posture was epic! It was mind-blowing! From that point on, we could no longer perform routine checkups the same way. Now, we had a choice and the responsibility to refer patients to experts trained in this area or learn more to help our patients ourselves. I chose to keep learning and continued my intensive training ever since.

NOSE BREATHING IS DOPE

Probably the most important thing I've learned is how essential breathing through our nose is!

Nasal breathing is essential for good health—it's actually how nature designed us to breathe. In fact, babies can primarily only breathe through their noses until about three months old. However, a mix of internal and external environmental factors often shifts this natural pattern, turning nasal breathers into mouth breathers, which can lead to various long-term subtle and not-so-subtle physical and neurological issues.

External factors like air pollution, household allergens, pets, and food allergies can cause nasal congestion. Other influences, like bottle-feeding, tongue and lip ties, pacifiers, and even food textures, can directly or indirectly block nasal passages and encourage mouth breathing. Since the first and second industrial revolutions, about 300 years ago, these environmental changes have impacted how our genes are expressed. As a result, we see narrower faces, recessed chins, and crowded teeth—a reflection of less-than-optimal growth and development in modern humans. Check out the video https://youtu.be/OdbV4HH4Sgk for more information.

Over time, it seems like everyone has "needed" braces. Unfortunately, with our modern desire for quick fixes, orthodontists often choose to pull teeth to align the remaining teeth to fit the mouth, rather than expanding the mouth to allow the teeth to naturally align. This means that instead of letting teeth grow into their genetically determined, site-specific positions, external forces are used to rearrange them.

I consider myself blessed to have had doctors who took a different approach, believing in helping the body reach its full growth potential with supportive tools rather than altering what nature intended. This is why my treatment, which began early during mixed dentition (when baby and adult teeth are both present), took three years. Early intervention provided a key opportunity to guide my growth properly.

MOUTH BREATHING IS NOT DOPE

Did you know?

The tongue acts like a scaffold for the roof of your mouth (palate), which is also the floor of your sinuses. During breastfeeding, a baby presses the breast tissue against the palate to draw milk. This natural action doesn't just provide food—it also applies pressure that stimulates stem cells to grow bone, expanding the nasal passages, sinuses, and the entire oral cavity. This natural development provides for proper breathing space.

People who chew loudly often do so because they are mouth breathers, although new studies have shown that swallowing and breathing can partially overlap. For mouth breathers who struggle to breathe through their nose, eating—especially chewing and swallowing—can be challenging. When you chew with your mouth open to keep breathing, it causes loud chewing sounds. This habit also prevents food from being chewed thoroughly, placing extra strain on the digestive system.

Nasal breathing is the most efficient way to breathe because it slows down our breathing rate and allows us to take deeper breaths. Together, these factors help ensure that our body can take in more oxygen and release carbon dioxide more effectively, maintaining a healthy balance.

When someone hyperventilates, we have them breathe into a paper bag because they breathe very quickly and often through their mouth. This rapid breathing causes them to lose too much carbon dioxide too fast, which can lead to feelings of dizziness, lightheadedness, and anxiety. Breathing into the bag allows them to re-breathe some of the carbon dioxide they just exhaled, helping to restore the balance of gasses in their body. This is why nasal breathing is so important—it helps prevent hyperventilation in the first place by keeping the breathing rate slower and more controlled.

Nasal breathing naturally filters and warms the air before it reaches our lungs. Thanks to the turbinates (bone structures in the nasal passages), the air also mixes with nitric oxide (NO), which is produced in our sinuses. Nitric oxide has amazing benefits:

- It relaxes airway muscles and boosts lung blood flow, helping the lungs absorb more oxygen and reducing the heart's workload.
- It helps to keep our airways open wider.
- It helps prevent pathogen growth (infection) in the airways.

Even more fascinating, nitric oxide serves as a neurotransmitter, sending signals that support brain function, such as regulating proteins—all from the nose!

Mouth breathing dries out the mouth, leading to inflammation of the tonsils and adenoids, creating a perfect environment for bacterial infections like strep throat, as well as bad breath and congestion. Simply breathing through the nose at night can actually help prevent bad breath!

Not-so-fun Fact: Adenoidectomy and tonsillectomy are common surgeries to remove the adenoids and tonsils, but these procedures often provide only temporary relief. The symptoms usually return because the root cause— mouth breathing—isn't addressed.

Mouth breathing triggers a fight-or-flight response, which is necessary for survival in emergencies but harmful as a constant state. Chronic mouth breathing can lead to neurological, endocrine, and metabolic disorders over time, as well as many other health challenges.

Mouth breathing ultimately causes sleep deprivation, which is an underlying cause of neurological disorders. A study led by Dr. Karen Bonuck on 11,000 children over a six-year period supports the argument that the children diagnosed with ADD and ADHD were nothing more than sleep-deprived. https://youtu.be/vRXkic9ftQU.

RESTFUL SLEEP?

Looking back to my story, none of us, including my brother himself, knew that he actually saved my life.

Shortly after beginning treatment, I stopped bed-wetting. At the time, it was thought that I had finally outgrown this common childhood issue. Today, I know better. I know that this condition, medically known as nocturnal enuresis, is directly related to dropping oxygen levels at night caused by either obstructive sleep apnea or another breathing disorder syndrome.

When a child (or adult) stops breathing at night, the brain shifts into a fight or flight response and reroutes the oxygen from some organs to save itself. One of the organs that is most often affected is the bladder, which loses control of maintaining its function of urine retention, and through bladder pressure, urine is released. Bottom line, there is a direct correlation between sleep apnea in children and bed-wetting. Who knew?!

SNORING

Wait! Do you hear the rumble? Do you hear the puffing? Does it startle you? Does it startle your bedmate? Yup! You guessed it. That scary noise is sometimes so loud. You believe the person is possessed. And often, they sleep right through it. It's called snoring.

The Oxford Dictionary defines snoring as "the action or fact of making snorting or grunting sounds while asleep."

Nearly everyone snores once in a while, but for some people it's a chronic problem that may need special attention. Snoring occurs when airflow passes through the relaxed tissues in our nose and throat and causes the collapsed tissues to vibrate as we breathe. It's a red flag that must be evaluated to make sure no sleep apnea or other breathing disorder is occurring.

Sleep apnea is a condition where a person's breathing stops and starts while they sleep. This often happens because the airway gets blocked when the nose and throat muscles relax. One of the most common contributors to this is mouth breathing. When someone breathes through their mouth, the pressure created as well as the position of the tongue make it more likely for the airway to collapse. This can cause snoring and gasping for air, interrupting sleep and leading to fatigue during the day, high blood pressure, irregular heart rhythms, and a whole array of health issues.

This condition is not only observed in adults. It is increasingly observed in children, starting in infancy. Early intervention is paramount.

You'll often read or are told that snoring is more common as we age because muscle tone decreases, causing our airway muscles to be less resilient. It's important to understand that other factors can be involved as well. Structural features, tongue ties, constricted or underdeveloped jaws like I had, and nasal obstructions can all affect adults and children equally. In addition, chemically induced airway muscle relaxation can be caused by the consumption of alcoholic beverages and certain medications.

If you or any loved ones, regardless of age, exhibit signs of sleep apnea such as snoring or gasping for air while sleeping, I urge you to reach out to an airway-focused dentist, pediatrician, or physician. It can be life threatening for some, and for others, setting them up for a poor health trajectory through their lives.

THE SKILL

WHAT CAN YOU DO TODAY TO HELP WITH NASAL BREATHING?

1. Become aware of how you are breathing at any moment of time. Like, right now. Is your mouth open? If yes, and if you can, close your mouth and remind your brain to start breathing through your nose. What about the people around you? What do you notice?

2. Reprogram our brain by training our nasal muscles and nerves through specific breathing exercises.

The process involves inhaling through the nose and exhaling through the mouth. As discussed earlier, there are essential functions that happen in the nose that are not triggered during mouth breathing. Exhaling through the mouth allows more carbon dioxide to be released from our lungs and promotes more oxygen uptake at the next breath.

One fun fact I've learned is that alternate nostril breathing stimulates opposite parts of our autonomous nervous system. Right nasal breathing activates the sympathetic nervous system and is performed to increase arousal and energize our emotional state which means increasing happy feelings; it increases cognitive focus and decreases mind wandering. On the other hand, left nostril breathing stimulates the parasympathetic nervous system which decreases blood pressure and heart rate and alleviates a state of stress.

There are a few nasal breathing techniques aiming at improving oxygen uptake and increasing energy while putting your body in deeper relaxation. The three main exercises I teach my patients are the **Coherent**, the **Ujjayi**, the **4-8-8** breathing technique. Each one of them is roughly performed for five minutes at a time.

The Coherent technique:

You can do this while sitting and relaxing, going about your daily tasks such as doing dishes, or even while walking. Breathe slowly in through the nose for five to six seconds and exhale out through the mouth for five to six seconds. Find your rhythm and create your cycle. It should not be uncomfortable. Repeat for five minutes.

Dr. Richard Brown, a psychiatrist at Columbia University has used this method to treat his patients. Regardless of the severity of their condition, he would have them breathe two seconds in through the nose and two seconds out through the mouth for ten minutes, and would then increase it to four-second cycles a few weeks later and eventually to five to six-second cycles. His results were phenomenal!

The Ujjayi technique:

This follows the same method while tightening the throat muscles and making noise from the throat while exhaling. It may sound weird and awkward, but so what? This technique simulates a deep humming sound and allows for even deeper relaxation than the coherent method.

The 4-8-8 (modified from 4-7-8 technique):

My favorite method is the 4-7-8 technique developed by Dr. Andrew Weil and slightly modified by James Nestor to 4-8-8 to give it a more rhythmic cycle. This slight twist may have made me more compliant with the exercise and, therefore, has become my number one choice, a favored breathing technique that provides deep relaxation, best done at bedtime for a good night's sleep.

Inhale through the nose for four seconds, hold for eight seconds, and exhale through the mouth slowly for eight seconds. Repeat for a total of five minutes. This technique builds up the carbon dioxide level, which triggers more efficient use of oxygen.

EVEN MORE YOU CAN DO

These are all great exercises to get you in the habit of nasal breathing. Sometimes, they're all you need. But if you have nasal congestion or blockages, facial structures that don't readily allow this flow or other conditions, you must work with a knowledgeable practitioner to help you properly address these.

If you're somewhat adventurous, you can look into trying mouth taping. It's using a gentle piece of surgical tape to hold your lips closed, which encourages you to breathe through your nose instead.

I strongly recommend good nasal hygiene before bedtime and using nose strips along with mouth taping. This method has been shown to reduce inflammation of the adenoids and the tonsils, often avoiding the need for surgery.

It would also be very beneficial to find a myofunctional therapist, a specialist who can design a set of exercises to help you, and especially your children (because the earlier you start, the better), to have better tongue positioning and airway strength, and less default to mouth breathing. After all, the tongue is your nature-made retainer!

Let us begin the process of recapturing our lost reflex of nasal breathing, an essential part of being healthy for life.

"Use it or lose it"!

Okay, now I'm going on a nature walk, a breath break. I often use breath exercises when walking. I love taking advantage of a beautiful autumn day to replenish, and today, my grandson is waiting!

Remember—practice makes perfect!

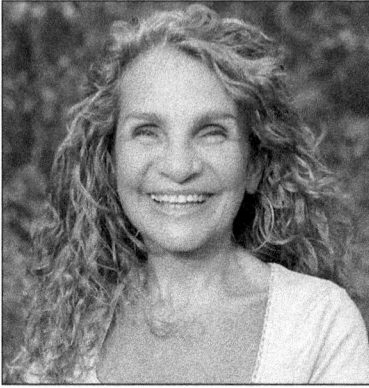

Dr. Najwa Jaber is a highly respected dental health expert with over two decades of experience in comprehensive family dentistry and specialized care for sleep apnea and breathing-related disorders. Known for her patient-centered integrative approach, Dr. Jaber emphasizes the vital connection between oral health and overall wellness, especially in the context of sleep health. A graduate of New York University, she has extensive training in advanced dental techniques, including focused expertise in sleep apnea management and TMJ dysfunction.

Dr. Jaber is dedicated to patient education, helping individuals understand how oral health impacts everything from heart health to quality sleep. Dr. Jaber's passion for patient education drives her to actively engage with her patients on subjects such as the links between sleep apnea and cardiovascular risk, the role of oral appliance therapy in treating breathing disorders, the importance of early intervention in children, and the impact of nutrition on dental resilience. Her work has earned her accolades for excellence in both patient care and clinical innovation.

In her chapter, *Breathless – Recapturing the Lost Reflex of Nasal Breathing*, Dr. Jaber explores how dental health can influence systemic health, with particular emphasis on sleep apnea and breathing. She provides readers with insights into how addressing sleep apnea through dental intervention can significantly impact overall health, empowering individuals to improve their wellness through targeted oral health strategies. Dr. Jaber's expertise and commitment to holistic care make her a powerful advocate for the role of dental health for lifelong wellness.

Dr. Jaber's multicultural background exposed her at an early age to communities deprived of adequate care and a healthy environment. Fluent in English, Arabic, and French, and conversant in Farsi, Spanish, and Wolof (Senegalese dialect), Najwa's ability to communicate with vast and varied audiences expands her natural sense of compassion across diverse cultures.

Dr. Jaber is the proud mother of three loving children and their growing families. When not in the office, she enjoys cooking and hosting family and friends; she also enjoys nature walks and hiking, the beach, dancing, and traveling.

Connect with Dr. Jaber:

Website: www.smileforme.com

Facebook:

https://www.facebook.com/SmileForMeLLC

https://www.facebook.com/najwa.bahsoun

PERSPECTIVE

Open minds save lives.

PERSPECTIVE: AN OVERVIEW

Perspective is everything. It's the lens through which we view and interpret everything in life, and it plays a crucial role in how we approach health and well-being.

While it's not one of our official "forgotten foundations" of health, its the often unseen force that impacts them all. Perspective shapes our mindset, priorities, actions, and decisions. The way we approach health depends on perspective—whether we see it as a burden or an opportunity, an unyielding set of rules or a flexible framework for resilience and growth.

Focusing too narrowly, like driving while only seeing the road ahead, blinds us to the bigger picture—the trees, hills, and opportunities around us, or the deer about to dangerously cross our path. Yet zooming out too much can obscure important details. Standing before a forest, we might admire its collective beauty but miss the fruit growing on one tree, the birds chirping in a nest, or the roots connecting the ecosystem. A healthy perspective helps us balance the big picture with the essential details.

A flexible, open mindset allows us to grow, connect, and find better solutions. Conversely, strict dogma can trap us in unhelpful patterns. Health, like life, demands a dynamic and open approach. That's why "open minds save lives."

In *Healthy for Life*, perspective is key to integrating the five foundational pillars of health—nutrition, environmental exposures, nervous system regulation, fitness and movement, and sleep. Shifting our perspective lets us reframe health as a journey of discovery rather than a rigid destination. It empowers us to challenge norms, embrace small changes, and build habits that align with our unique needs and values.

CHAPTER 26

UNLOCKING POTENTIAL

THE POWER OF CURIOSITY

Mariah Ramundo

MY STORY

Ring, ring. "Hello?"

"Hi, Mariah. Daycare is on the line, I'll transfer them."

"Okay, thank you."

Deep breaths, Mariah, deep breaths. Don't cry.

"Hello?"

"Hi Mariah. You have to come get your son. He has a fever, and he can't return until you have a doctor's note and he's fever-free for 24 hours." *Click.*

I froze, staring at a picture of my sweet baby boy on my desktop while watching my inbox continue to flood with emails.

What am I doing here?

Who am I?

What is my real title; am I a mom or am I an employee?

How can I remain a top-performing employee and a mom at the same time?

Why does this keep happening to me?

What am I doing wrong?

I lived in a pressurized system since returning to work after my maternity leave.

I didn't even have time to think about being a wife, daughter, friend, sister, aunt, niece, or any other "job title."

How could I? I had zero bandwidth to even take care of myself.

This routine weekly call from daycare meant that I was out of work again for at least another 48 hours. I closed my office door and collapsed in tears. I took some more breaths and then called my pediatrician's office to schedule yet another appointment.

This visit was different, though. I looked at the walls as I was walking out, where they promoted the upcoming flu clinic and health insurance facts for payments. I searched for a sign that said something like this: "Are you struggling with anxiety and depression?" I walked further down the hall before checking out, looking for more signage that would promote some kind of community or resource for the new moms who are struggling to keep it all together. *I wish they had some kind of hotline posted so I could talk to someone.* I wasn't suicidal, but I was not okay. And, at the same time, a part of me didn't want to admit openly that I felt like I was failing as a parent. I didn't feel like myself anymore.

My project deadlines and revenue goals at work were now at risk of not being met, but they secured my job and paid our mortgage, daycare, medical bills, and household overhead. Sleepless nights were my norm as my child remained chronically unwell. Our pediatricians have no answers and only prescriptions, laugh at me for asking questions, and still collect their payment before I leave their office each week.

I must not be the only one going through this, am I?

Some colleagues in our office ganged up on me and reached out to my VP behind my back to comment on how I am "never in the office" so that it's noted on the agenda for my upcoming weekly one-on-one. I worked hard to keep my composure and manage it all without complaining so that from the outside looking in, from female colleagues who do not have children—or children with special needs or chronic health challenges—it probably really did look like I was just "signing off" and leaving for the day. I couldn't speak up about what was going on, or I would break down. I wasn't ready to be that vulnerable with people who seemed to lack genuine curiosity, compassion, and empathy to consider that maybe there was something more serious going on.

I pretended every day that my life was perfect while inside, and in reality, it was falling apart. I was falling apart.

I put my own basic needs (eat, sleep, drink, exercise) on the back burner to prioritize this new schedule of "urgency" that ran my life for years.

I had my scheduled one-on-one with my VP. I wasn't nervous to share what was going on because he always created a safe space for me to expand on the truth of what was happening so that trust could remain strong. At the time, he didn't know that some of the females in the office struggled with infertility. Saying to them, "You will understand when you have kids," wasn't an appropriate response to support me. I struggled to find a way for them to consider exercising some sort of emotional intelligence into my situation. I dislike excuses, though, so I never speak up about the severity of my situation to this team, and I continue to suffer in silence.

As the primary wage earner in our home, and with my outside sales job being the "flexible" job compared to my husband's, I was always the parent responsible for these weekly daycare calls, pick-ups, and doctor's visits.

My husband had just taken a new job, and he had little to no paid time off. He worked in a highly controlled test laboratory where he needed his sleep, or any teensy, tiny human error could potentially blow up him and the lab—literally. He was not an option to lean on in the middle of the night or during the day—I cared too much about his safety to risk losing him. I continued to suffer and couldn't find a way to share the depth of anxiety and depression I felt.

I finally decided to "quit" my pediatrician. I strongly disliked their approach of continuing to mask symptoms with medication (that had short and long-term side effects) while also following their recommendations to rotate Tylenol and Motrin weekly to help manage his pain and fevers. As a loyal person, a part of me judged myself for leaving their practice, yet I knew "nothing changes if nothing changes."

He was born healthy; how has this changed so much in just a short period of time?

I spend days and nights doing research and outreach to qualify the next best pediatrician. Our former office was "the best of the best," according to all of our family and friends.

Our new pediatrician immediately suggested an evaluation because she's concerned about some of his developmental delays. I worry now that this is directly correlated to the side effects—known and unknown—of the medications the previous office prescribed. I scheduled for the therapists to visit our home and evaluate our son. They suggested he qualified for services. *Finally*, I thought.

A month passed, and we got paperwork in the mail stating we were denied services. I was totally confused again. My heart's racing. *They must've made a mistake.* I called them directly to inquire about the obvious error made in the transfer of the information shared during the evaluation to the letter that denied us any and all services. The woman who answers the phone apologizes and states, "Although he could benefit from services based on his evaluation, we are short-staffed, and there are many more children who need our services as a priority. When he's another year older, you can have the school evaluate him."

How can they discriminate based on their workplace staffing challenges? I'm still so confused.

I fully understand the demands required for prioritizing urgent and more serious cases, but adjusting the results with messaging that feels everything but inclusive felt completely unethical. *Back to the drawing board.*

At times, I truly felt like I was penalized for using my growth mindset to help him through challenges so that he wasn't as "bad" as the other children. I inquired about the names of therapists since the two women who visited the house shared the specific areas of growth for him, and I was prepared to pay more out of pocket to get the support we needed. They had none.

How is this even possible? I feel like I'm in the Twilight Zone.

And, when I reached out for support from our trusted immediate and extended family, I was criticized and judged for labeling him. They were more concerned about how they looked, having a family member with a label, versus helping me find the right people to get our son the resources he needed. A common response was, "You'll be okay; I got through it with no support, and my kids turned out fine." Or, they would act as though these sensory challenges, developmental delays, and constant healthcare concerns and crises were normal and said he'd "grow out of it."

At this point, we are struggling to pay all of our bills on time with the accumulated medical bills. My husband at the time even doubted the chaos I was living by questioning my concern about the number of doctor visits and prescriptions, asking me to prove it.

How is this my life right now?

Why is everyone in denial?

Everything seems so transactional around me.

I'm genuinely confused and concerned that no one hears me when I do speak up. No one is listening, nor does anyone seem to care.

Am I not communicating properly?

Or am I asking the wrong people for support?

I was a pro at managing it all on my own up to this point. Some days, I wore my burnout as some sort of badge of honor; it feels better to not sulk in sadness. It was definitely a title I worked hard for by then. *Fake it until you make it, right?*

This anxiety, stress, and burnout continued for years. It became my lifestyle, and although it constantly kept my nervous system tense, I still felt like I was progressing—until I wasn't. This kind of stress and burnout is not sustainable. What happened next was inevitable.

I scheduled a visit with my primary care physician and broke down. She prescribed me an anti-anxiety medication. I took one dose and turned into a total zombie and suddenly lost my zest for life and my passion. I had no motivation or inspiration for anything anymore. This didn't feel right at all. It definitely did its job, as I didn't care to care anymore. How scary that was for someone who feels so deeply!

I called the office, and they scaled it back to the lowest dose, which I even cut in half—still a zombie.

I go back to the familiar, what I know worked in the past. I decide to discontinue the medication and carry on with my normal routine—yes, the burnout one.

I got extremely run down, and with the lack of sleep, nutrition, and high level of stress I experienced, one of my closest clients actually asked me at a meeting, "Are you high? Your eyes are so bloodshot."

"I'm exhausted," I replied. "I'm burned out. I don't sleep. I'm up all night with my son. And I have no idea how to help him get better."

Deep down, I intuitively knew the two-inch stack of medication receipts from the pharmacy wasn't actually getting to the root cause of the issues.

There has to be a different way. Why do I have to keep defending myself?

I read about mindfulness in my late-night research, and it wasn't until I listened to a podcast quoting this phrase (specifically) that I started to change my thoughts from *Why does this keep happening to me?* to *What is this teaching me?*

I used this perspective to shift my awareness. I moved from a victim mindset (not downplaying any of the trauma that happened) to one that is more positive and comes from a position of strength. This phrase reminded me that one day I'd be on the other side of this, able to pay forward these lessons I was growing through to others in a big way. Adding a future goal to help more people and parents trapped in this same kind of trauma felt inspiring and very purposeful to me.

"The things that excite you are not by chance; they are connected to your purpose."

~ Danielle Laporte

This mindset shift allowed me to move from a first-person perspective to a third-person perspective. It allowed me to detach from the reality of my stressful situation and see it through a different lens. During this shift, I remembered this profound piece of evidence: anytime our body is stressed, our nervous system gets hijacked, and the decision-making part of our brain automatically disconnects.

Is this why I haven't been able to figure it out yet? I feel like I am getting closer to answers.

That third-party view, or what's called dissociation, could be considered negative, yet I felt it was my superpower. I worked extra hard to stay at this 30,000-foot high view now. With this strength back online, I tapped into creative ways to manage stress and burnout more effectively and efficiently. Breakthroughs happened.

Next, I researched local therapists.

I didn't want a traditional therapist. I Googled different keywords based on the outcomes I was desiring, where there'd be an interdependent relationship with tools and techniques provided to work on in between sessions. I wanted a coach-type of energy where there was mutual trust, respect, and accountability. I wanted a strengths-based therapist that focused on strengths and well-being and not just challenges. And I found one.

My positive psychology therapist changed my life.

I was so grateful to have finally found a safe space where I could vulnerably share my experiences and start to develop an awareness of how I was managing so well on my own. She provided research along with many tools, books, journal prompts, podcasts, and meditation, as well as additional mentors, groups, and communities of moms who had grown through similar experiences. There were sound therapy, yoga recommendations, and more. She even introduced me to the CEO of Wholebeing Institute, where I enrolled to learn how to bring my strengths—supported by their credentials—to the world. I created a new life rich with healthy habits that supported my overall well-being: spiritually, physically, emotionally, intellectually, and relationally. I learned how to take care of myself first with these new healthy habits versus pouring from an empty cup– my old norm.

I think I found myself again. This version of me wasn't the same as the Mariah I once knew, though.

Harnessing curiosity and these brand-new healthy habits have allowed for many more very meaningful and valuable introductions into the holistic healing community. Curiosity led me to the best doctors, practitioners, and experts and helped me to finally feel connected, seen, and heard. This new mindset helped me no longer suffer in silence. This new network that I organically and tirelessly cultivated through curiosity was finally able to get to the root cause of our labels and reverse every single health issue we have had. The psychological implications of our stories and experiences have also been reversed.

Curiosity truly unlocks potential.

"When you know better, you do better" is the Maya Angelou quote that allows me to forgive myself and others for what we didn't know.

I now completely trust in the timing of my life.

THE SKILL

"Growth mindset is the psychology of success"

~ Dr. Carol Dweck

Are you ready to go from post-traumatic stress to post-traumatic growth?

Instead of the traditional psychology model focusing on what's *wrong* with you, positive psychology focuses on what is *right* with you. We take a strengths-based approach to optimizing the human potential. Positive psychology is the science of happiness and includes research on how habits can either help us or hurt us.

It's actually very common that we need to hit rock bottom to change our habits. And, having an awareness of what our habits are is how we start changing them.

Our habits do include our thoughts.

Our thoughts can be limited through a fixed mindset, or they can be abundant through a growth mindset.

The primary way to shift from fixed to growth is through curiosity. Curiosity is the key positive psychology strength (and habit) that physiologically rewires the brain and changes who we are completely. It's what allows for post-traumatic growth.

Who we are entering trauma is completely different from the person we are when we're growing through it and when we're on the other side of it.

Research shows that applying your strengths can increase confidence, resilience, happiness, and health. The VIA Character Strengths Test is a widely utilized, scientifically validated assessment tool that helps people thrive in both their personal and professional pursuits.

My number one top strength of "love of learning" is exactly how I thrive in this lifetime. It's how I build resilience. And, as it relates to my story, my innate passion for doing research and interviewing many different practitioners, therapists, and doctors is why we're able to authentically thrive now. My story is directly connected to my life›s purpose to empower others to share their story in a safe and confidential space where there is no judgment, shame, criticism, or fear of retaliation or rejection. The closest person to an expert is someone who lived (grew) through it.

Reducing the number of people who suffer in silence is more of a global movement that positive psychology directly supports.

Below is a step-by-step process on how to immediately start creating a growth and strength-based mindset that will positively transform your life and the relationships around you.

"Whether you think you can or you think you can't, either way you're right"

~ Henry Ford

STEP ONE

Tap into curiosity to explore what your top character strengths are here: www.viacharacter.org

STEP TWO

Become aware of your top strengths (we are born with all 24). Once you're intentional about seeing these in yourself, look to spot others with these strengths also. For example, when talking to your child, "Wow, I noticed your *bravery* when you jumped over the log—great job!"

STEP THREE

Dedicate intentional time after reading this book to tune into the chapter, thought leader, and/or story that resonated the most. What we see in ourselves, we often see in others, so you may naturally gravitate to a story that demonstrates your top character strengths.

STEP FOUR

Go for a walk and/or journal with only curiosity, imagination, and creativity about what your life could look and feel like if you were to work with this expert to support where you're feeling burnout.

STEP FIVE

Use your growth mindset to schedule time with them to explore how they could shift your life from a state of survival to one that's more thriving. Remain curious and ask questions.

What you are not changing, you are choosing.

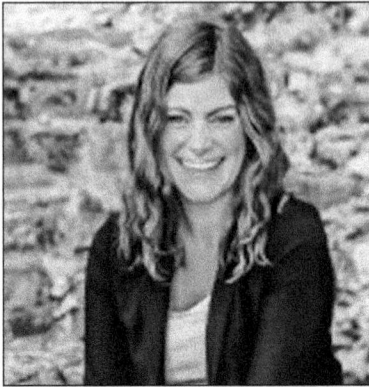

Mariah Ramundo is a dedicated strategic and visionary thought leader who is passionate about unlocking potential in individuals and businesses through a holistic, strengths-based approach. With over 16 years in corporate sales, leadership, and human resource management, she combines deep professional experience with a commitment to personal growth and well-being. Mariah's work integrates positive psychology with practical tools, fostering environments where resilience, growth, and success thrive.

Through her coaching sessions, workshops, and retreats, Mariah empowers others to connect with their innate strengths and purpose, creating pathways to meaningful transformation. Her approach is rooted in both evidence-based methods and an intuitive understanding of each client's unique journey, making her guidance both effective and personalized.

Connect with Mariah:

Website: https://www.mariahramundo.com

CONCLUSION

"Just as ripples spread out when a single pebble is dropped into the water, the actions of individuals can have a far-reaching effect."

~ The Dalai Lama

Healthy for Life isn't just a book—it's the start of a transformative journey for you, your family, and ultimately the world. Throughout these chapters, we've laid out, in five pillars, the forgotten foundations of health, and within each, important skills to get you started: *Nutrition, Environmental Exposures, Regulation of the Nervous System, Fitness and Movement, Sleep, Repair, and Recharge.* We've also shared essential paradigms for navigating the world around us: *Proactive Prevention and Perspective.*

You have the power to make a difference and give children their best chance. As adults, we're in the unique position to guide the younger generations, and we're the ones who will shape their future health, for better or worse. We need to be the example they see, not just the advice they hear.

Nothing is one size fits all. We are complex, coordinated beings, a remarkable intelligence working in harmony within ourselves and our surroundings. The solutions to our health problems aren't one-size-fits-all, and no single strategy will solve everything.

You don't need to have all the answers or get it right every time. Just take what resonates, start where you are, and keep moving forward. Even on days when life feels overwhelming, or progress feels slow, your journey is inspirational in and of itself. By building these forgotten foundations in your life, you're not just improving your health—you're setting up future generations for a better, brighter path.

One More Quote–another essential perspective:

I'll leave you with one more quote. It may help you think about how to stand your ground in a world that's always trying to pull you in a million different directions.

"Compromise where you can. Where you can't, don't. Even if everyone is telling you that something wrong is something right. Even if the whole world is telling you to move, it is your duty to plant yourself like a tree, look them in the eye, and say 'No, you move.'"

~ Peggy Carter, Marvel Cinematic Universe

This is more than just a rebellious attitude—it's about recognizing that when it comes to your health and the health of your family, you don't need to follow the crowd. You don't need to accept shortcuts, compromises, or habits that don't serve you. When it comes to the health of you and your loved ones, you are in charge—and sometimes, that means planting your feet firmly in the ground and saying, "No, you move," to the unhealthy choices that society is constantly pushing our way.

Healthy for Life! This is a movement— to bring health back to its roots. Your journey toward resilient health begins now, and it starts with one small step and one heartfelt guiding voice! What will it be?

ACKNOWLEDGMENTS

Healthy for Life would not have been possible without the support, dedication, and passion of many remarkable people. My heartfelt gratitude goes out to each and every one of you who made this journey inspiring and impactful.

To the Brave Healer Productions publishing team:

Laura Di Franco, thank you for your awesome vision of bringing these powerful collaborative books to life. Your signature quote, *"Your words will change the world if you're brave enough to share them,"* has empowered me and the whole author team to do just that—to share our heartfelt stories and the wisdom we've been fortunate to learn in our respective life journeys. Kelly Kaschula, you've been so warm and helpful. Thank you for your diligence. Dino Marino, thank you for your amazing talent and patience in helping craft a design that truly captures the soul of this project.

To the incredible team of co-authors:

Some of you signed on without a second thought just because I asked. You so warmly made it clear (each in your own way) that you know me, both as a doctor and a mother, trust me, my intentions, and my vision, and want to join forces. Thank you more than words can say, from my heart, for being friends and colleagues by my side always.

Others, who are now my new friends, thank you for also trusting me and my vision. I've already had the privilege to learn so much from you by reading your stories and getting to know you. You're contributions to the book and the *Healthy for Life* movement moving foreword are integral.

To some "wing people" in my life:

Amanda Carpenter, for saying, "Hey, I know you've always wanted to write a book; you should contact Laura." Literally, without you, this powerful and unmatchable collaboration would not have happened. Thank you for looking out for me always.

Adria Rothfeld, my sounding board through this entire process. Thank you for keeping me in flow (and sane).

Armin Brott, the wisest writer and amazing editor. You will always be my trusted advisor.

Stephen Cohen, that one insightful, fortuitous phone call from Amy Levine Cohen became one of the most pivotal calls of my life. I'm blessed to have you as an ally.

Yael Lieberman, my right hand, thank you for holding down the fort as amazing as always, including while my attention was on this book.

To my family members:

My brother Ari, you are an inspiration. When you put your mind to something, you get it done. In my high school yearbook, I wrote, "I only yell at you because I love you." That holds true, but now it's "I only nudge you because I love you."

My in-laws, Yair and Lea, who have raised a wonderful family. Yair passed away recently in no small part from medical mismanagement. This fuels my determination even more. My mother-in-law Lea, it means so much that you appreciate and embrace my medical advice, and I am so happy to always help you how I can.

My daughter-in-law Genie, you're now under my watch as well. This only adds to the knowledge I seek and the heartfelt care I have for your best life and health.

To you, the reader!

Thank you for taking the time to hear from us. I wish you the resolve, knowledge and skills for you and your loved ones to be Healthy for Life!

For additional resources visit our website:

www.HealthyforLifeBook.com

www.ingramcontent.com/pod-product-compliance
Lightning Source LLC
Chambersburg PA
CBHW070056030426
42335CB00016B/1914